Piet G de Boer | Robert Fox

Changing patterns of lifelong learning
A study in surgeon education

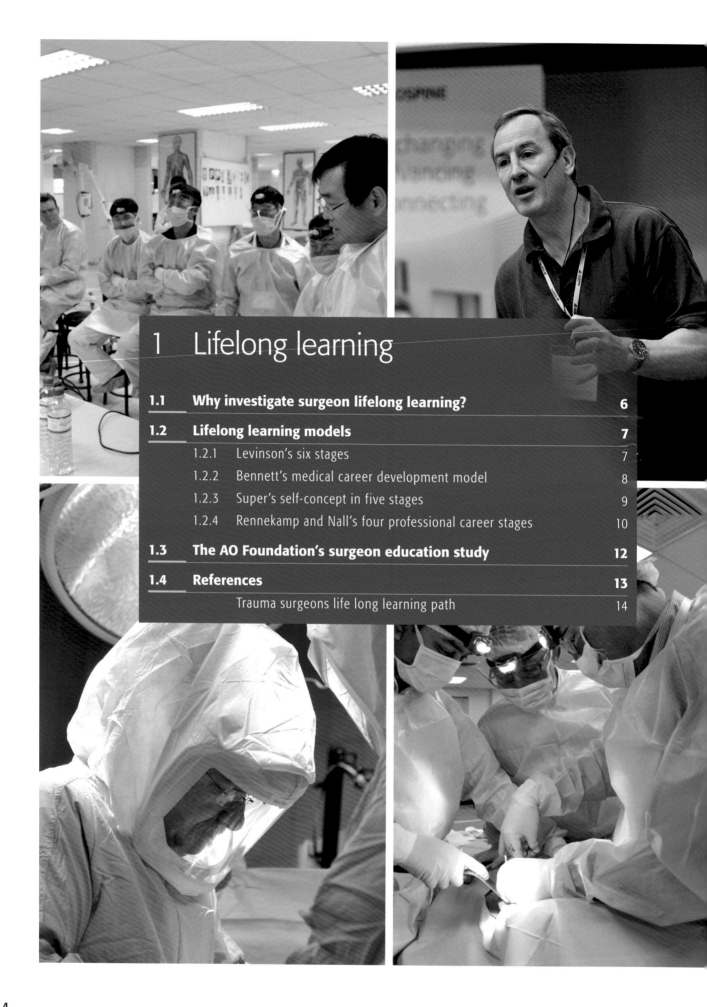

1 Lifelong learning

Chapter 1
Lifelong learning

From residency to retirement, continuing learning is part of each stage of a surgeons' career because it is instinctively associated with better patient care, improved outcomes, and the application of new technology. Nearly all practicing surgeons, educational leaders, and policy makers can agree that lifelong learning is a necessary component of a successful surgical practice.

The old concept that a surgeon ceases formal learning after completion of residency is obsolete. Surgeons now require to access education throughout their practicing career. Lifelong learning is a standard requirement for all surgeons and not merely the territory of the academic [1,2].

Surgical practice is rapidly evolving and standards of practice are changing. Patients, employers, and governments expect surgeons to keep themselves up to date and practice to an acceptable level of competence. Increasingly surgeons are also required to document the steps taken to ensure that their practice is current.

Highly developed medical systems, such as in the United States, have defined requirements for health professionals to maintain their professional status. This in turn has led to pressure from staff to access adequate educational opportunities to maintain their professional status. Developing countries have very different systems of maintaining professional standards, varying from none to highly sophisticated systems. Very little is known about the requirements for postgraduate medical education outside the English-speaking world and even less about the systems in place to meet this need.

1.1   Why investigate surgeon lifelong learning?

Suboptimal care has been part of medicine since its inception and remains an issue for surgeons and patients alike. Traditional professional attitudes which led to hiding or denying mistakes have completely altered in the last 30 years. Health care systems and professionals are now focused on reducing errors. The problem has been addressed by a variety of approaches such as critical incident reporting, systems analysis and audit as well as postgraduate medical education. Unfortunately, each approach has met with limited success [3–6].

Part of the explanation for the failure of some postgraduate medical education to improve patients outcomes may lie in the lack of understanding of how surgeon's needs may vary with their age and experience. Everyone who wishes to help surgeons change their behavior through education needs to know how surgeons as "learned professionals" are using learning over the course of their practicing lives. What experiences do surgeons have and how do these relate to the different ways that learning may occur? What are the surgeons' responses to the transitions and transformations they experience in their lifelong commitment to quality care?

In order to grasp the complexities and challenges surgeons experience as they move through their careers, we need to understand and explain how and why changes occur. We need to be able to understand the ways that surgeons manage these changes. We also need to know how learning contributes to the different stages of a surgical career. Finally and most importantly we need to know what educators can do to help surgeons grow more competent and less likely to make errors that impact their patients.

The criteria laid down by major specialty societies, professional regulatory bodies for reaccreditation, professional organizations, and medical colleges focus on lifelong learning. Yet these organizations have little real evidence as to the stages of development that medical professionals pass through or the implications of those developmental stages for lifelong processes of education. This knowledge gap is most profound in terms of surgeons and their careers. In order for educators to provide appropriate services and to be able to assist in the learning process, what is needed is an understanding, not only where we ought to be in terms of lifelong learning opportunities, but also where we are today.

One way to understand how and why learning changes over the career of the surgeon is to engage in traditional research that looks at stages of development, such as conducting surveys or mining demographic data related to the learning activities of physicians and surgeons at different stages of their career. The problem with this approach is that such quantitative methods only work when you have a deep understanding of the processes to be studied enabling the researcher to assign numbers and to measure accurately the differences that exist among surgeons at different stages of their career. A high level of precision is needed so that the numbers become meaningful rather than meaningless. Without such a precise understanding there is very little hope that the solutions derived from such a study would be practical and useful.

Complex phenomena, such as the transitions that surgeons make from stage to stage throughout their career and the impact of these transitions on lifelong learning, can only be understood through a process that involves in-depth exploration—in this case, studying actual experiences of real surgeons as to how their careers progress and their reflections on how learning and education play a role. Such a study gives an understanding of actual processes and suggests potential directions to target focused change.

This study was developed with the idea that by understanding over 100 surgical careers in-depth, we could present a representation of the pathways that are characteristic of orthopedic surgeons as they progress through the stages and transitions that characterize their career. We could understand how these changes affect their learning processes and the activities they engage in to improve surgical care. Such an in-depth exploration using rigorous interview procedures should reveal and portray accurately the stages surgeons experience and the transitions that accompany those stages as they move through their career.

1.2   Lifelong learning models

The idea of moving through a developmental process is neither new nor revolutionary. Humans advance through different phases of life—it is an intuitive journey. We have always described children as moving through stages, and even Shakespeare in *As You Like It* described seven stages of life. In fact there is an historical body of literature about how adults progress through stages of development. These investigations provide a framework for approaching the question of how and why surgeons pass through different stages and transitions on their career pathway.

1.2.1   Levinson's six stages

The first formal account of the various stages in adult development dates from 1977 with the publication of a book by Daniel Levinson entitled the *Seasons of a Man's Life* [7]. Levinson's description was groundbreaking because it was the first theory to describe development that occurs throughout the adult years, as opposed to childhood.

Levinson based his model on biographical interviews with 40 American men aged between 35 and 45. They worked either as biology professors, novelists, business executives, or industrial laborers. The model therefore resonates most strongly with men in the developed world and has less relevance to non-western and developing societies. It should also be noted that the model does not apply to women. Levinson published a second book called *Seasons of a Woman's Life* nearly 20 years later [8]. Each subject was interviewed between 6 and 10 times and each interview lasted between 1 or 2 hours.

Levinson described certain stages in adult life and differentiated two types of stages—stable and transitional periods. A stable period is defined as the time

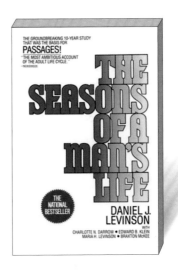

when a person makes crucial choices in life, builds a life structure around these choices, and seeks goals within this structure. A transitional period is defined as the end of a stage and a beginning of a new stage. The transitional periods were times of stress and during transition the presence of a mentor or older teacher was a positive influence in guiding the person through the obstacles in their life path.

The six stages of adulthood as described by Levinson:
1. **Early adult transition (17–22)**—men leave adolescence/school and make preliminary choices for adult life.
2. **Entering adult world (22–28)**—men make initial choices in love, occupation, friendship, values, and lifestyle.
3. **Age 30 transition (28–33)**—changes occur in a man's life structure either as a moderate change or more often after a severe and stressful crisis.
4. **Settling down (33–40)**—the subject establishes a niche in society in both family and career accomplishments. Men are expected to think and behave like a parent and so face a more demanding world where more is expected from them.
5. **Midlife transition (40–45)**—the subject starts to question his life structure. It is usually a time of crisis. Neglected parts of self (talents, desires, and aspirations) seek expression. Men become involved in trying to leave a legacy and this usually forms the core of the second half of their life.
6. **Entering middle adulthood (45–50)**—choices must be made, a new life structure formed, and the person commits new tasks.

The midlife transition phase became popularized as the "midlife crisis" but from the point of view of medical educators looking at lifelong learning, Levinson's most relevant comment may be:

"As long as life continues, no period marks the end of the opportunities and the burdens of future development."

Levinson's work was the first to suggest that there were distinct and definable stages in a man's life. Mature readers of this monograph will probably be able to identify with some if not most of the life stages he describes. His work however resonates mainly on the personal and the emotional sides of life. Can his model be applied to career progression in surgery and does an understanding of it aid medical educators in making their educational offerings more effective?

1.2.2   Bennett's medical career development model
In 1989 Continuing Medical Education expert Nancy L Bennett examined the career pathways of physicians because she felt that, "An understanding of the professional and personal development of health care professionals is an essential component for providing continuing education" [9]. She found that Levinson's model did not fit certain aspects of a doctor's life:

"Doctors start their first independent job close to the time of the age thirty transition without having been involved in some of the decisions of early adulthood. Their personal lives, including marriage and children may have been put on hold. There can be a sense of being off schedule behind peers in other professions." Specifically, the midlife transition that in Levinson's model is often stressful, coincides with a time when a surgeon is moving into a stable practice.

Bennett went on to describe a three-stage model of career development in medicine beginning after the completion of resident training.

"First, physicians start by breaking in to medicine, testing out the ways they will fill the role of a physician. They formulate their ideas about how to practice medicine in this first step out of training. There is a shift from the sense of practice in training with extensive backup to a new level of responsibility for patients. New resources must be found, and the right times for their use requires much thought. Some physicians try several roles to find the one, which seems to provide the best fit between real and ideal visions of medicine.

In 3 to 5 years, after gaining some experience, physicians fitting into medicine tailor their lives based on experience, a more stable practice, and a need to look again at what has evolved in their careers. Confidence from experience may be used to break away from the traditional practices within the community, to specialize, or to think again about the usefulness of standard procedures. Physicians as a group become less like each other in response to individual views of how medicine and a personal life fit together. For some, the changes were very dramatic, impacting on all aspects of life. For others there is an adjustment to refocus in smaller ways.

Bennet's three stage model of career development in Medicine:

1 Trying to conform

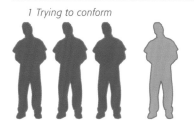

Lastly, physicians getting out of medicine think about retiring. This stage often takes a long period of time and is accompanied by high levels of stress. The decision to relinquish patients, many of whom have grown with the physician, is very difficult. Those getting out worry about their standing within the community, their vulnerability to malpractice, and how their colleagues think of them.

2 Trying to become different

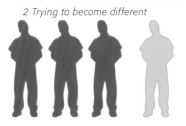

Bennett's three stages could be summed up as trying to conform, trying to become different, and trying to leave. She concluded by stating that more research was needed to understand the career pathways of doctors. She felt that if medical education was to be more effective than it must be tailored to the requirements of the learners and if this were to be done then we must understand the effects of age and state of development on learning and performance of doctors.

1.2.3   Super's self-concept in five stages

3 Trying to leave

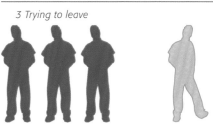

In 1990, Donald Super was one of the first career theorists to describe certain distinct career development stages [10,11]. His work was also based on a large number of interviews, and its core theory is that the development of an individual within his career is related to the notion of self-concept. Self-concept is basically how individuals picture themselves and has been defined as, *"The constellation of self-attributes considered by the individual to be vocationally relevant"*. This picture includes the individual's abilities, personality traits, values, self-esteem, and self-efficacy.

He proposed five stages of career development:
1. **Growth**—characterized by the individual's first introduction to the world of work.
2. **Exploration**—individuals gather more specific information about themselves and the world of work.
3. **Establishment**—individuals act on the information gained during their exploratory phase by matching their interest and capabilities to their occupation. During the establishment stage, individuals are concerned with career advancement in their chosen occupation. They are trying to establish a stable work environment with a potential for growth and the opportunity for promotions.
4. **Maintenance**—individuals are concerned with maintaining their present job status. During this phase individuals may change organizations.
5. **Disengagement**—individuals are focused on developing a self-image and a self-concept that they are independent of and separate from work.

Donald Super's work was mainly focused on the corporate world. The career stages he described overlap those described by Bennett in the world of medicine. Super's stages one and two—growth and exploration—correspond closely to Bennett's stage one, fitting in at the start of a surgical career. Super's stages three and four—establishment and maintenance—correspond to Bennett's stage two, differentiation. Finally, Super's stage five—disengagement—corresponds to Bennett's stage three, retirement.

1.2.4 Rennekamp and Nall's four professional career stages
In 1993, psychologists Roger A. Rennekamp, and Martha A. Nall, tried to define career stages to those engaged in the professions [12,13]. They built on the 1997 work of Dalton, Thompson, and Price [14]. They defined four stages in a professional's career.

The entry stage
The entry stage corresponds to a time in a professional's career where the individual first enters the profession or a new job within the profession. The entry stage is characterized by some psychological dependency. The central motivators for professional development at this stage include attaining the foundation skills required to do the job and understanding the organization's structure.

They suggested that the motivation for professional development at the early stage included:
a. Understanding the organization's structure, function, and culture.
b. Attaining basic level technical skills.
c. Giving relevancy to previous training.
d. Exercising creativity and initiative.
e. Moving from dependency to independence.
f. Building relationships with professional peers.

This definition of the entry stage corresponds to residency and the first few years of independent practice when applied to the career of a surgeon.

The colleague stage

The colleague stage is characterized by an individual trying to build at least one area of expertise for which he or she is noted.

The motivations for professional development at the colleague stage include:
a. Developing an area of interest.
b. Becoming an independent contributor in problem solving.
c. Developing a professional identity.
d. Gaining membership of the professional community.
e. Moving from independence to interdependency.

This definition of the colleague corresponds to the stage in a surgeon's career where he or she develops a specialist interest.

The counselor stage

The stage is characterized by individuals taking on leadership roles particularly in professional associations. They accomplish most of their work through others and have extensive networks both within and outside an organization.

The motivations for professional development at this stage include:
a. Acquiring broad-based expertise.
b. Attaining leadership positions in professional circles.
c. Developing networks with other organizations.
d. Stimulating thought in others.
e. Counseling other professionals.
f. Developing coaching and mentoring relationships.

This definition of the counselor stage corresponds to that stage in a surgeon's career when he or she becomes a senior surgeon within his institution.

The advisor stage

The final stage is that of the advisor. These individuals play a key role in shaping the future of the organization by supporting promising people, programs, and ideas. The adviser often has a regional or national reputation and a comprehensive understanding of the organization. Their motivations for professional development include:
a. Becoming involved in strategic organizational planning.
b. Achieving the respect of others in the organization.
c. Engaging in innovation and risk-taking.
d. Achieving a position of influence.
e. Sponsoring individuals, programs, and people.

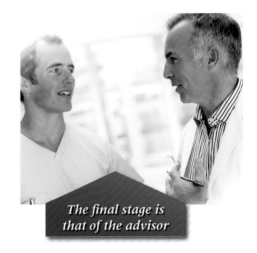

The final stage is that of the advisor

Although this definition of the advisor stage may resonate with many surgeons, most trauma surgeons do not aspire to achieve such a position.

These models of the stages of life and careers suggest that individuals go through definable stages and transitions but none relate directly to the career stages of surgeons. All these studies originate from the United States and very little is known how these stages might differ throughout the world. To investigate these unanswered issues this study was initiated and sponsored by the AO Foundation.

1.3   The AO Foundation's surgeon education study

The AO Foundation [15] is a medically guided nonprofit organization led by an international group of surgeons specialized in the treatment of trauma and disorders of the musculoskeletal system. It offers affiliated surgeons and operating room personnel (ORP) global networking opportunities and knowledge services. It provides educational courses globally and these events attract over 30,000 surgeons and nurses from 57 different countries each year.

The primary study questions were:
1. Do trauma surgeons undergo clearly defined stages in their careers? If so, what are those stages?
2. Why do surgeons access education? What is their motivation to learn?
3. Do surgeons change the reasons why they look for education depending on their career level?
4. Do surgeons differ in their choice of educational channel depending on their career stage?
5. Do current educational offerings meet those educational needs and if not where are the gaps and how could they be filled?

Secondary study questions were:
1. How has surgical training changed over the years?
2. Does the preference of educational channel depend on age as well as stage of career?
3. How are the various educational channels (books, journals, mentoring interpersonal relations, courses, meetings, Internet) currently used and what are the trends?
4. What is the relationship between trauma and orthopedics both in training and with regard to career pathway?

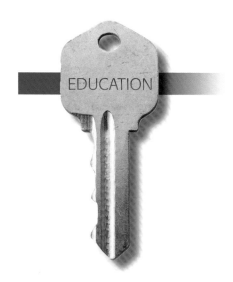

To investigate these questions a study was carried out which is presented in this book. The core of the study consisted of a series of in-depth interviews with 100 international surgeons. It was a qualitative study to give practicing surgeons an opportunity to voice how education had affected them at various stages of their careers.

A quantitative study was not possible or desirable for two reasons. Firstly, very little is known about this subject. Initial investigation of any area of scientific interest should first define what needs to be examined, and to do this open-ended questions are required. Secondly, a quantitative study would not allow surgeons to tell their own individual stories, reflecting the richness and depth of a surgeons' practicing life.

It may be that things were missed or not asked. However, the stories taken together give us a better idea about how to structure more effective and responsive educational systems.

Vignettes will be found throughout this monograph to illustrate the surgeon's stories. It is hoped that some of these vignettes will resonate with those readers who are practicing surgeons themselves and illustrate the huge variability of practice environments and the surgeon's response to them.

This study was undertaken to provide educationalists with a good and fundamental understanding of the way orthopedic surgeons progress from surgical residency to retirement. Understanding the transitions and stages that surgeons go through provides a basis for developing more in-depth learning opportunities. Explaining how surgeons progress through their careers allows verification of learning needs, and establishes reasonable and well grounded approaches that nurture the educational development process.

Such understanding also helps surgeons at each stage of their career to adjust and manage their lifelong learning needs in terms of patient care. Educational events and material can be more precisely targeted if these processes are understood, and as a result the education provided may be more likely to change surgical practice to the benefit of the patient.

1.4   References

1. **Schön D** (1983). *The Reflective Practitioner, How Professionals Think In Action.* Basic Books. ISBN 0465068782
2. **Kolb AY, Kolb DA** (2005). Learning Styles and Learning Spaces: Enhancing Experiential Learning in Higher Education. *Academy of Management Learning & Education;* 4(2):193–212.
3. **Kumar S, Stenebach M** (2008). Eliminate US hospital medical errors. *Int J Health Care Qual Assur;* 21(5): 444–71.
4. **Wolf FA, Way LW, Steward L** (2010). The efficacy of medical team training: improved team performance and decreased operating room delays: a detailed analysis of 4863 cases Ann. Surg; 252(3): 477–485.
5. **Willis CD, Stoelwinder JU, Lecky FE** et al (2010). Applying composite performance measures to trauma care. *J Trauma;* 69(2): 256–62.
6. **Mahajan RP** (2010). Critical incident reporting and learning. *Br J Anesthesia;* 105(1):69–75.
7. **Levinson DJ** (1978). *Seasons of a Man's Life.* New York: Ballantine Books.
8. **Levinson DJ** (1987). *The Seasons of a Woman's Life.* New York: Ballantine Books.
9. **Bennett NL** (1990). Theories of Adult Development for Continuing Education. *J Cont Educ Health Prof;* 10(2):167–175.
10. **Super DE** (1957). *The Psychology of Careers: an introduction to vocational development.* New York: Harper and Row.
11. **Super DE**. Self concepts in vocational development in DE Super (ed), Career development: Self concept theory New York; College Entrance Examination Board.
12. **Rennekamp RA, Nall M** (1994). Growing through the stages: A new look at professional growth. *Journal of Extension;* 32(1).
13. **Rennekamp RA , Nall M.** Professional growth; a guide for professional development. Lexington: *University of Kentucky Cooperative* Extension Service.
14. **Dalton G, Thompson P, Price P** (1977). The four stages of professional careers: A new look at performance by professionals. *Organizational Dynamics;* 6(23).
15. **AO Foundation** – http://www.aofoundation.org.

Trauma surgeons life long learning path
(AO Foundation model life long learning path)

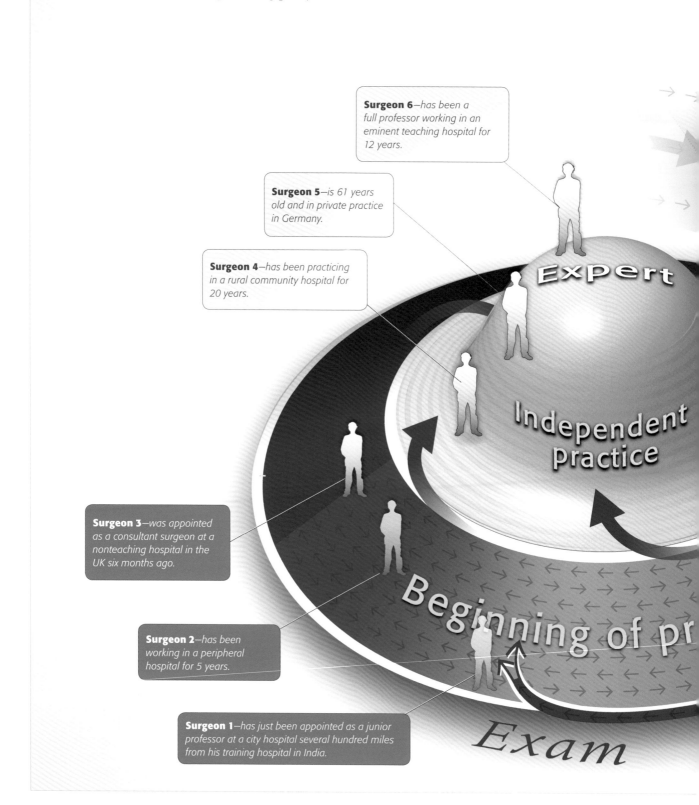

Surgeon 6—has been a full professor working in an eminent teaching hospital for 12 years.

Surgeon 5—is 61 years old and in private practice in Germany.

Surgeon 4—has been practicing in a rural community hospital for 20 years.

Surgeon 3—was appointed as a consultant surgeon at a nonteaching hospital in the UK six months ago.

Surgeon 2—has been working in a peripheral hospital for 5 years.

Surgeon 1—has just been appointed as a junior professor at a city hospital several hundred miles from his training hospital in India.

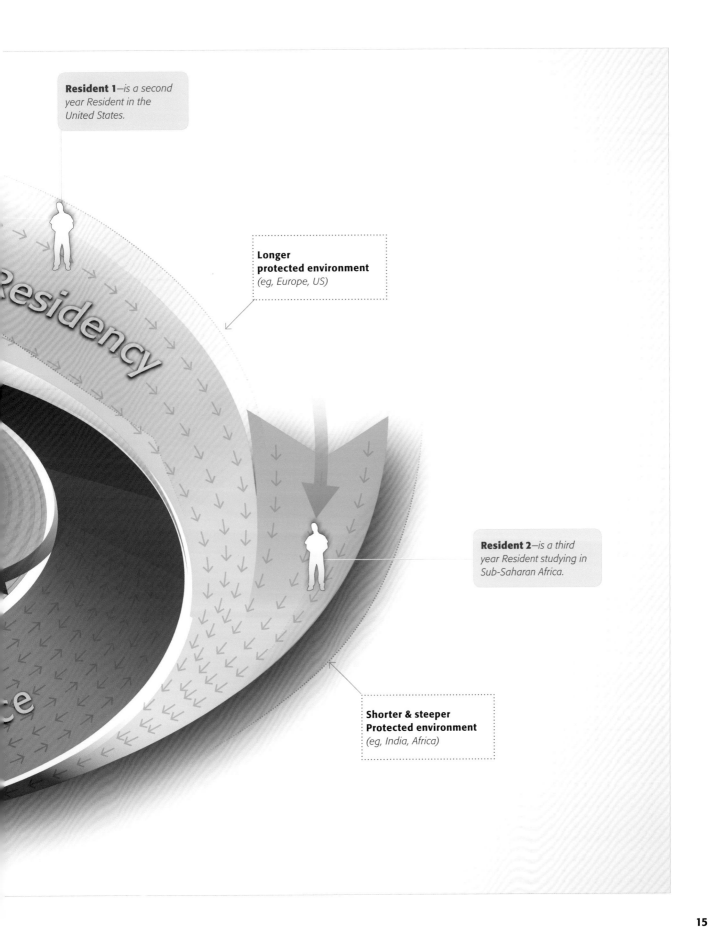

Resident 1—*is a second year Resident in the United States.*

Longer protected environment *(eg, Europe, US)*

Resident 2—*is a third year Resident studying in Sub-Saharan Africa.*

Shorter & steeper Protected environment *(eg, India, Africa)*

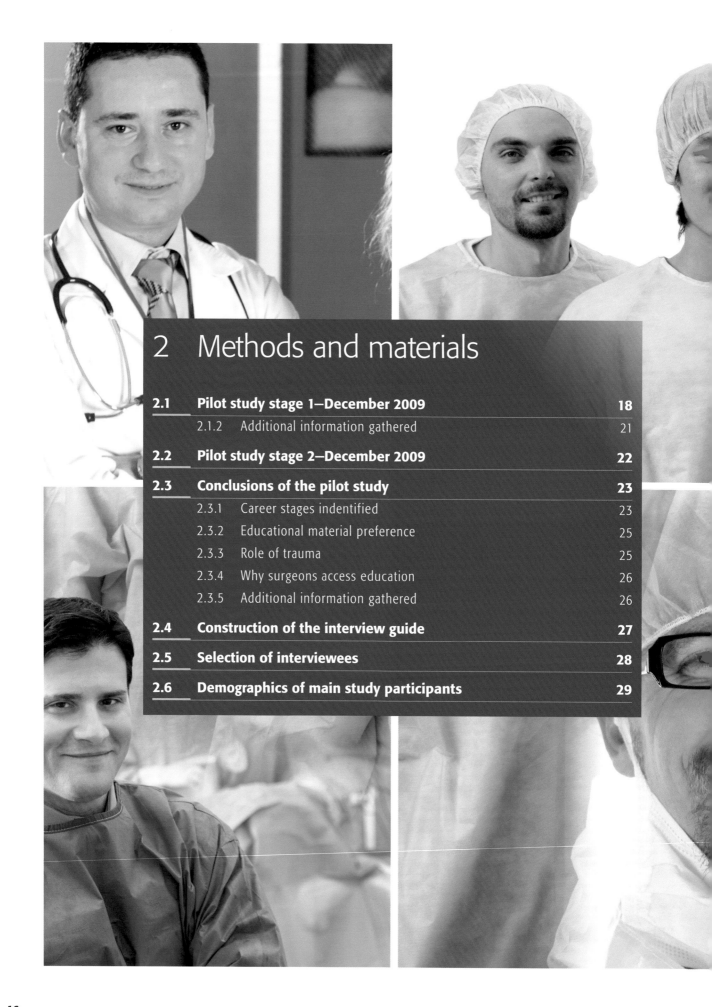

2 Methods and materials

Chapter 2
Methods and materials

The lifelong learning Study intended to examine the career stages of surgeons and their educational needs and preferences. Design of the main study was informed by data gathered during a two-staged pilot conducted in December 2009 at AO Davos Trauma Courses.

Because the aim of the lifelong learning Study was to explain a process and not to test or verify an existing theory the grounded theory approach of sociologists Barney Glaser and Anselm Strauss was used.

The pilot group consisted of 47 surgeons who were initially interviewed in both focus groups and individually before the main study instrument in accordance with grounded theory's iterative study design was set up. The pilot study involved a limited number of surgeons and open-ended questions were asked. Analysis of this preliminary data informed the design of the next cycle of data acquisition allowing the creation of an interview template that would be used in the main study.

The pilot study was carried out in two parts. The first part consisted of interviews carried out with focus groups. The second part consisted of more in-depth one-on-one interviews with surgeons. The pilot involved course participants and faculty attending an educational event—the AO Davos Trauma Courses—and was carried out in December 2009. The pilot study asked the following questions:

1. Did surgeons recognize that there are different stages in their career and were they able to describe these stages?

2. Were surgeons able to describe the reasons why they access education in their practice? If so, what are the main reasons why they access educational help?

3. Were surgeons able to clearly articulate what forms of educational help are of most use to them at their current stage in their career? If they were, what are their preferred educational channels?

4. What are the current CME mandatory requirements for them in their own practice? What is the effect of these regulations on their practice/educational requirements?

2.1   Pilot study stage 1—December 2009

At the opening session of every course taking place in the first week of the two-week event course participants were invited to attend an early morning focus group to be interviewed. The course chairman made this invitation orally. Participants were offered the incentive of a €50 voucher that could be redeemed for textbook purchase. Three hundred and fifty surgeons were invited.

Twenty-six participants attended two focus group meetings. The surgeons interviewed were of varying degrees of experience. Thirteen of these 26 were experienced surgeons with more than 10 years postresidency experience. Four surgeons had between 5 and 10 years postgraduate experience. Five surgeons were in the first 5 years of independent practice and four surgeons were still in residency training.

Experience of interviewees

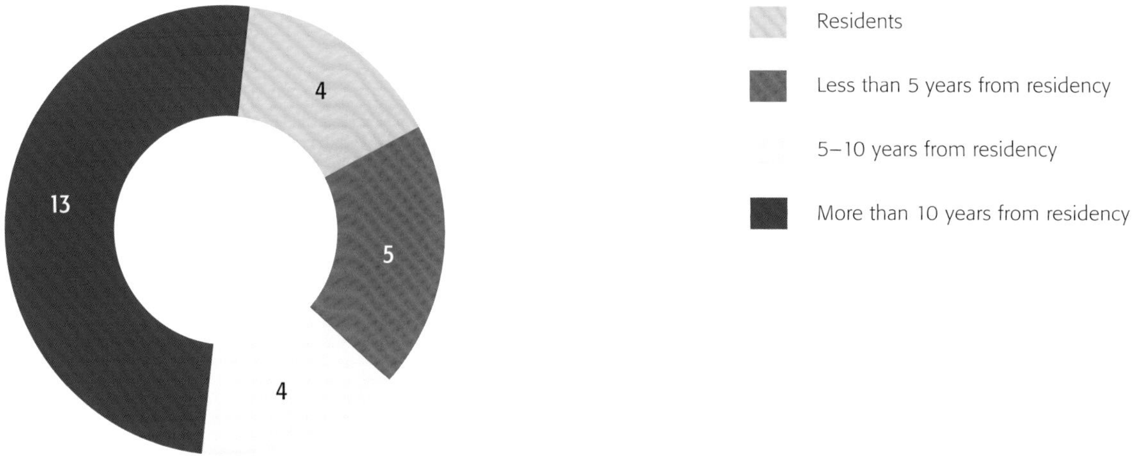

Residents

Less than 5 years from residency

5–10 years from residency

More than 10 years from residency

Figure 1 Career experience of participants in stage one of the pilot study.

The surgeons interviewed in the focus groups came from all parts of the world. Half of the attendees at the focus groups came from the Asia Pacific area, but within this group there were no representatives from the People's Republic of China. The rest of the attendees at these focus group meetings were evenly distributed between Europe, North America, South America, and the Middle East.

Origin of interviewees

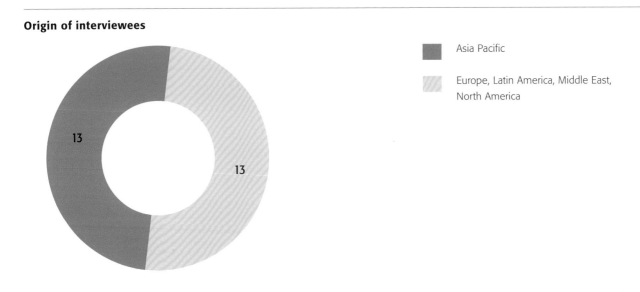

Asia Pacific

Europe, Latin America, Middle East, North America

Figure 2 Geographic origins of participants in stage 1 of the pilot study.

The focus groups lasted 50 minutes. Attendees were asked to describe the career structure for a trauma surgeon within their own country and where they felt they were in their career. They were asked why they currently access educational help and why they had done so in the past. They were also asked what their preferred channel of access to educational material was. The questions asked were open-ended **and no attempt was made to channel discussions within a predetermined framework.**

These focus group interviews showed clear answers to the four study questions.

1. Did surgeons recognize that there are different stages in their career and were they able to describe these stages?
Surgeons could identify a clear career progression structure within their own countries and were able to say where they were in their career pathways. They recognized that they had gone through and would continue to go through different stages in their professional development. Career pathways did differ in different parts of the world especially when the period immediately after completion of residency was considered.

A surgeon from India described a career structure reflecting gradual change from residency to independent practice. *"I did a three year residency program which led to me getting my Masters. After that I stayed on in my teaching hospital progressing from Associate Professor to Assistant Professor. It was a gradual change, getting more independence and responsibility. After 5 years I left and set myself up in private practice. I treated anything that came in through the door. I soon realized that here was a huge demand for joint replacement surgery so I got myself a fellowship in the UK to learn the trade. I am now the local expert in joint replacement and have recently accepted a part-time post in my local government teaching hospital so I can pass on my knowledge."*

A more dramatic change from residency into independent practice was part of this surgeon's career from the United States. *"Immediately after I finished my residency I went straight into private practice. It was a hard transition having to take call. Although I had done a lot of independent surgery as a senior resident it was a very stressful time. At that time arthroscopic surgery was becoming more and more popular so I specialized in that and sports medicine. I guess I was largely self-taught but now I reckon I am up there with the best."*

2.   Were surgeons able to describe the reasons why they access education in their practice? If so, what are the main reasons why they access educational help?

All the surgeons interviewed could clearly describe the reasons why they accessed education. Overwhelmingly surgeons access education if they have a clinical problem. This was true for surgeons of all grades of experience no matter what country they came from.

A typical response came from a surgeon from the Ukraine. *"Why do I look for education? Usually, it is because I come across a problem I don't know how to solve. For years all we had were some old Russian textbooks and it was hard to change. Now we have access to the Internet and more chances to travel so I can find solutions to my problems."*

3.   Are surgeons able to clearly articulate what forms of educational help are of most use to them at their current stage in their career? If they are, what are their preferred educational channels?

Surgeons accessed education in a huge variety of ways. These included:
- Personal interaction with colleagues/mentors
- Textbooks
- Journals
- Internet
- Meetings – hospital/local/national/international
- Formal educational courses

4.   What are the current mandatory CME requirements for them in their own practice? What is the effect of these regulations on their practice/educational requirements?

Although residency programs are well defined and usually characterized by an exit examination, CME requirements for surgeons in practice vary hugely from country to country. **In general, the surgeons interviewed did not feel that CME requirements were a major driver for accessing education.**

This surgeon from the United States expressed the majority view. *"Yes, CME is important but I can pick up my points very easily. If I go to an educational event I go because I need to find out how to treat my patients and not because I need the points."*

2.1.2   Additional information gathered

Because the interviews were open-ended certain other information was gathered outside the four study questions.

1. Few surgeons practice trauma exclusively. Most surgeons practicing trauma are orthopedic surgeons and their commitment to trauma is very variable. The majority of the orthopedic surgeons in developed countries regarded trauma as being only part of their job and their commonest career pathway as the surgeon gets older is to reduce trauma commitments. A job consisting purely of trauma surgery without elective orthopedic work is unusual. In developing countries, the amount of trauma work carried out by an orthopedic surgeon is much greater than the average orthopedic surgeon in the developed world; surgeons continue to treat trauma throughout their practicing lifetimes in these countries

Many surgeons felt that this was an advantage such as this surgeon from Sweden. *"Although we have our trauma experts most orthopedic surgeons carry out a mixture of elective orthopedic and trauma surgery. I think that the skills needed to carry out both specialties are similar and the two go well together."*

This UK surgeon gave an extreme view. *"No one in their right mind would carry out a pure trauma practice. There is no money in it and anyway most of it can easily be carried out by my residents. It's my aim to get out of trauma as soon as possible but my colleagues won't let me."*

This surgeon from Thailand gave a radically different view. *"Treating victims of trauma is the most important thing that we do. Although I now have a sub specialty of hand surgery I still feel that trauma is very important. It will always be part of my life as an orthopedic surgeon and I have a duty to ensure that my trainees do a good job."*

2. Who accesses education? Two surgeons clearly made a point that they felt that there were a group of surgeons in practice who did not access education in any significant way. *"It's not me and my practice that you should be interested in. It's the people who aren't here and the people who never go to courses. There are people practicing in my area who carry out very bad medicine and who never attend any educational courses or hospital meetings."*

3. Finances. Martin Allgöwer, a famous trauma surgeon, described the practice of trauma surgery at his investiture as a fellow of the Royal College of Surgeons in 1976 as, "The Cinderella of Orthopaedics". Trauma surgery is thought to be unfashionable and unprofitable in many developed countries. Many orthopedic surgeons seek to reduce their trauma commitment to maximize their income. For others, practicing trauma is very lucrative. *"You can only do trauma in a government hospital and a full professor's salary is a very good one. Also, you don't have any of the hustle of private practice.*

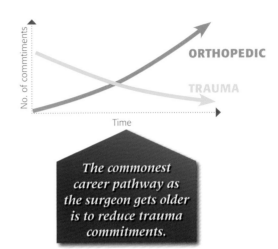

The commonest career pathway as the surgeon gets older is to reduce trauma commitments.

4. Orthopedic training. Orthopedic training is becoming more structured throughout the world. Most countries now have formal curricula and most have an exit exam. In developed countries, however, working time directives have resulted in less time being available to train orthopedics/trauma surgeons during their residency. This has resulted in residents leaving their periods of formal training with much less experience than in the past. *"I did about 36,000 hours of training during my residency. My current residents will do about 6,000 hours. I don't think these guys should be asked to act as consultants when they're appointed in the way I was. They just don't have enough experience to be able to cope."*

2.2   Pilot study stage 2—December 2009

Stage two of the pilot study involved open-ended, in-depth interviews with surgeons in all stages of their careers. The focus group data obtained in week one of the Davos educational courses allowed construction of an interview guide which was then tested on 21 orthopedic trauma surgeons attending the second week of the Davos Courses. At the start of every Davos course in the second week of the two week event surgeons were invited by their course chairmen to take part in interviews. They offered the incentive of a €50 voucher for educational books. Three hundred and twenty surgeons were invited. Each interview took approximately 30 minutes. A single interviewer conducted all interviews.

The interviewees included surgeons from all career stages. Three surgeons were residents in training, five were within their first 5 years of independent practice, five had between 5 and 10 years of independent practice, and eight had more than 10 years of independent practice.

Experience of interviewees

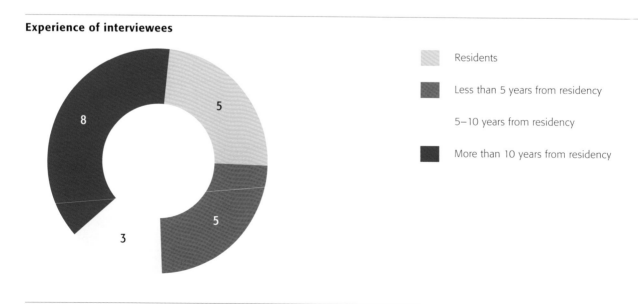

Residents

Less than 5 years from residency

5–10 years from residency

More than 10 years from residency

Figure 3 Career experience of participants in stage two of the pilot study.

Interviewees came from most geographical regions. Ten surgeons were from Europe, one from North America, one from the Middle East, and seven from Asia Pacific.

Origin of interviewees

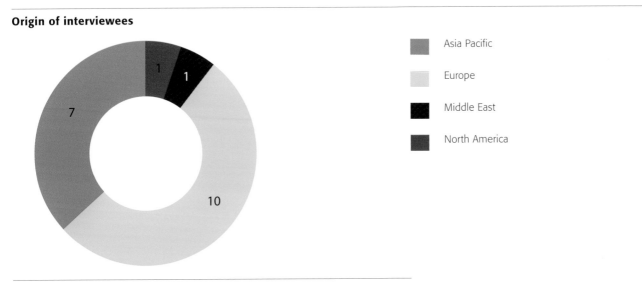

Asia Pacific

Europe

Middle East

North America

Figure 4 Geographic origin of participants in stage two of the pilot study.

2.3   Conclusions of the pilot study

The pilot study suggested that surgeons pass through distinct and definable career stages and that their educational requirements did change with their career stage. The variation in career pathways and the huge variety of educational preferences discovered suggested that a larger study should be carried out to more accurately describe both career patterns and the resultant educational requirements as they vary around the world.

2.3.1   Career stages indentified

All surgeons could identify clear career pathways within their country of practice and could recognize that they had been through different stages of their careers. Four career stages were described although there was considerable variation from surgeon to surgeon and from country to country.

Residency

All surgeons interviewed identified residency as a clearly defined period of training. Those senior surgeons who were interviewed and who were responsible for current resident education, commented on significant changes that had taken place in resident education, which will be discussed in a results section of the main study. *"Things are quite different now. When I was a resident it was see one, do one, teach one. Nowadays it is much better. My residents actually get supervised and we have a regular teaching program which we actually follow."*

Beginning of practice

This was the career stage that was the most problematic to define for the surgeons who were interviewed. Although all surgeons had a career change when they finished their residency, the nature of this change varied considerably. Some of the most senior surgeons went straight from residency into independent practice without any significant external support. Some of these surgeons found the transition to be extremely difficult. *"It was the most stressful time in my entire career. Although I was doing the same things as I had been doing in the last stages of my residency, somehow it all appeared to be very much more difficult."*

Other surgeons found this transition to be very easy. *"In effect, I had been operating independently since my second year residency. Moving to a consultant job was a very easy change for me to make."*

For others, the transition was not so abrupt. Some surgeons did not achieve independent practice at the end of residency, but took up postresidency posts within their training institutes still under the direction and supervision of a professor. The degree of their independence varied considerably. One surgeon from India commented, *"My boss just liked me to get on with things and not keep pestering him. He was always around though if I needed help."*

Although most of these surgeons subsequently went into independent practice, there are a small group of surgeons who never achieved independent practice, especially in Germany.

Developing specialization

All the surgeons interviewed either had specialist interests or wished to develop them. Fifteen of the surgeons interviewed said they either had or wanted to develop a specialist interest in orthopedics outside the field of trauma. The remainder either had trauma as their major interest. Some surgeons started to develop their specialist interests after a period of time in independent practice. Others started to develop a specialist interest while in residency.

Expert

The seven surgeons interviewed who had more than ten years of practice all considered themselves to be experts in their particular field. Three of these were specialized in trauma and the rest in differing fields in elective orthopedics.

2.3.2   Educational material preference
Although all the surgeons questioned regularly accessed educational material, there was a wide variation in their preferences.
It was unclear whether these preferences were related to their career stage, their age, or perhaps a mixture of the two, but the preliminary data collected from this survey suggested that more detailed questioning of a larger number of surgeons would be necessary to explore learning preferences in association with career stage.

Two surgeons, both of who were experts in their chosen fields had radically differing views *"I am a book person. I like to sit down, take my time and read. The only thing that is better than that is going to my national meeting and talking to my friends about the latest developments." "The Internet has revolutionised my life. I can access all the information I need at the touch of a button. Maybe I get too much information but at least it is up to date. I don't think books have much role nowadays."*

2.3.3   Role of trauma
There were significant geographical variations when the issue of how important trauma was to an individual surgeon's practice. In some western countries trauma is seen as a small part of an orthopedic career. *"Most of my colleagues in my hospital are desperately trying to work out how they can cut and eventually eliminate all their trauma commitments. It is of no interest to them and they usually get the juniors to do the cases for them."*

This is in contrast to the developing world, where trauma forms a very major part of an orthopedic surgeons' practice.

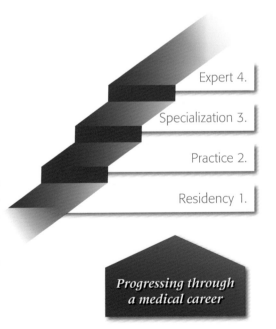

Expert 4.

Specialization 3.

Practice 2.

Residency 1.

Progressing through a medical career

2.3.4 Why surgeons access education

Although the main reason for accessing education was always a patient problem that the surgeon faced, other factors were also important. The role of changing technology seemed to be a fairly common theme and one US surgeon commented, *"There seems to be a new implant coming out every month. Although I guess most of them are a waste of space, you have to keep yourself up-to-date. If you don't, your patients will certainly tell you about it since they all have access to the Internet as well."*

A third reason for accessing education—the feeling that one's practice is getting out of date—was felt by one senior surgeon, who commented that his trainees had made him aware that his practice was quite outdated and that there were other newer technologies around.

2.3.5 Additional information gathered

Other points made by the surgeons, which were outside the main study questions included:

- The difficulty of getting access to formal educational courses—cost and the limited number of places available.
- The growing importance of fellowships as an add-on to formal residency.
- The fact that many hospitals are not keen on admitting trauma cases since it is not considered to be a revenue generator outside the United States.
- The socioeconomic pressures facing surgeons in the developing world
- The lack of good evidence-based solutions for treating common trauma problems.
- The competitive nature of progress in an orthopedic/trauma career.
- The geopolitical factors limiting surgeons' access to resources and education.

The surgeons who volunteered to be interviewed were clearly a self-selecting group. Their presence in Davos at an educational event showed that they had commitment towards their own education. By volunteering to take part in an early morning interview for the incentive of a 50 Euro book voucher, they showed themselves to be highly committed to an educational process.

This commitment of the doctors interviewed in this preliminary phase of the study is well illustrated by this comment from an Iranian surgeon who had struggled to get to the course *"Lifelong learning is about attitude. We must all learn to do our best. The problem is that the learning virus competes with the money virus and many people in the end become more preoccupied with money than any other aspect of their career."*

2.4   Construction of the interview guide

Data collected from focus groups and the individual interviews was used to create an interview script for the main study.

Because surgeons found it difficult to describe their career stages, the interview began by asking a series of relatively closed questions:

- How would you describe the current stage of your career?
- Do you recognize that there have been different stages in your career? If so, how would you describe them?

Because the pilot study had shown that various clearly defined learning modalities or channels had been used by surgeons, specific questions were asked about each of these learning modalities. The interviewee was taken through the various stages of his career and asked about every teaching modality at every stage in his career. The questions asked were:

- What role did people play?
- What role did literature play (eg, books, journals)?
- What role did formal educational events play?
- What role did Internet resources play(What resources have you used?)?
- What role did hospital meetings such as morbidity and mortality play?

In addition to these specific questions, two general questions were asked with regard to accessing educational resources at various stages of a surgeon's career. These general questions were:

- Can you remember particular methods of learning or characteristics of the stage X?
- When looking back, what method of learning was the most important to you during stage X?

Historical data, ie, what learning resources an individual surgeon used during previous stages in his career, is interesting and its analysis shows the evolution of teaching and learning methodologies with time. The purpose of this study, however, is to try to precisely define the current learning needs of surgeons and for that reason, a separate section was added at the end of the interview template relating to the surgeon's latest educational needs/experience. The questions asked were as follows:

- In the last year, have you made any changes to the way you practice surgery?
- What did you change and why?
- In what ways did learning play a role in changing your practice?
- What learning resources did you use?

The final interview template can be found in Appendix 1.

2.5   Selection of interviewees

A list of current members of the AO Alumni Association was obtained. The following information was available through this database.

- Name
- Email address
- Date of joining the organization
- Country of origin
- Gender
- Specialist interest
- Hospital
- Town of origin

The numbers of members identified were:

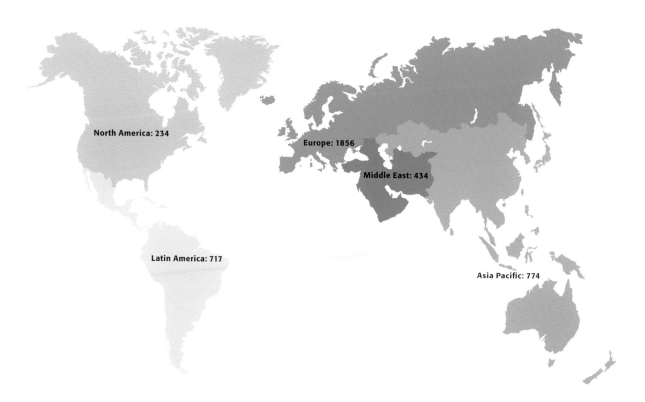

One hundred interviewees were selected from these 4015 names at random using the Google Random Number Generator. Interviewees were contacted by email. Those who responded to the email were contacted and appropriate interview times arranged by telephone.

Response rates varied considerably from region to region with language being a major barrier. Fifty-one interviews were carried out using this protocol. The remainder were carried out at educational events or by local surgeons interviewing their colleagues. These interviews were of course carried out in their native language.

2.6   Demographics of main study participants

One hundred surgeons from around the world were interviewed for this study. Thirty surgeons were residents-in-training, 17 surgeons were just beginning their post residency practice, 18 surgeons were becoming experts in trauma or another branch of orthopedics, and 35 surgeons were already acknowledged experts in their fields.

Experience of interviewees

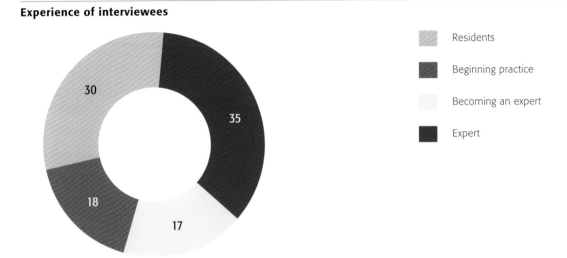

Residents

Beginning practice

Becoming an expert

Expert

Figure 5 Career experience of main study participants

Surgeons interviewed came from all regions of the world.
Thirty-three surgeons hailed from Europe, 19 came from North America, and 19 were from Asia Pacific. Seventeen surgeons came from Latin America and twelfe were from the Middle East.

Origin of interviewees

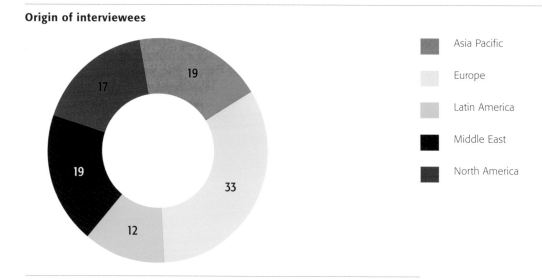

Figure 6 Geographic origin of main study participants.

The responses were collected and analyzed to identify the characteristics of each career stage, how it had changed with time and what the specific learning requirements of each stage were. The results are presented in the following chapters each of which is devoted to a particular career stage.

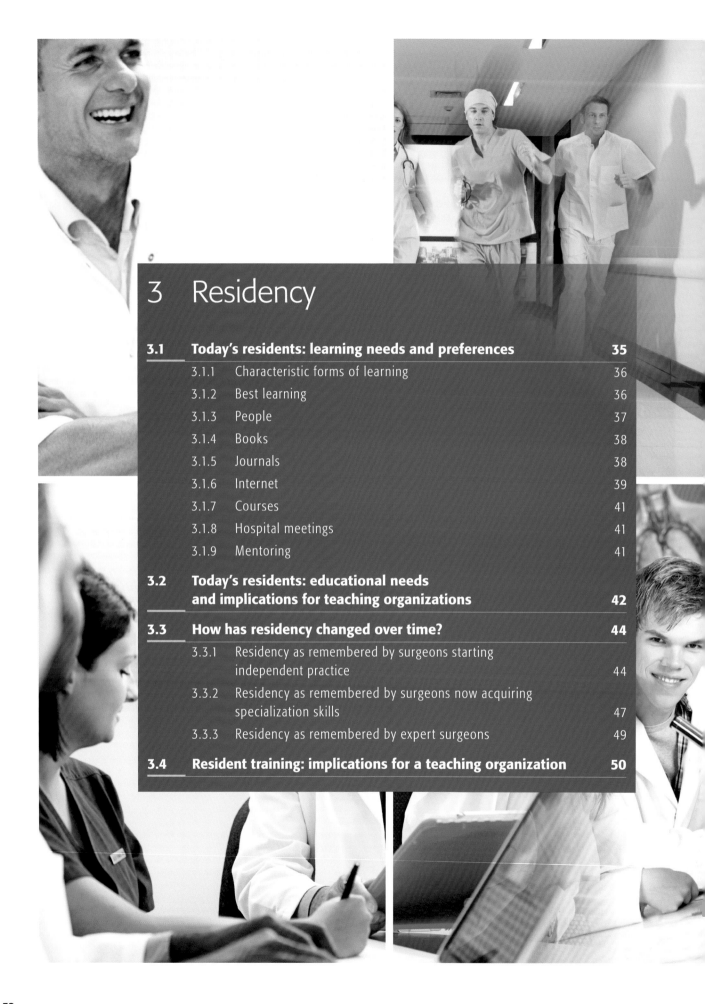

3 Residency

Chapter 3
Residency

Residency is the most easily defined stage in a surgeon's career. Yet, like most aspects of medical education, it has transformed over time. Teaching organizations must analyze the changes to stay competitive and anticipate the evolving needs of residents. Resident education is generally planned and executed by senior surgeons. If they fail to reflect on how things have changed since their own experience, educational offerings may reflect the senior's remembered needs rather than the resident's current ones.

Throughout the world residency is thought of as a period of supervised training leading to the creation of a surgeon who is capable of independent practice. Although there is total agreement about what residency should be, there are huge variations in the actual processes involved. This chapter looks at residency through the eyes of current residents and the memories of more senior surgeons who passed through residency training several years ago.

Entry into a training program is always preceded by a period of more general training usually carried out within the hospital system. This period of preliminary training varies between 1 and 4 years. **Entry into many formal training programs is competitive**, and in a few places, most notably Europe, surgeons do other non-specialist jobs for up to 3 years waiting to enter a formal residency program. Trainees who have to wait a significant time to enter formal residency programs characteristically take specialist educational courses such as the AO Principles Course before starting residency. Those with a shorter time before entry into residency training take such courses in the first or second year of residency.

Residents are predominantly male but the number of females entering orthopedic residency programs is increasing rapidly especially within the European Union.

It is generally agreed that residency training is now more formal and organized than it has been in the past. **Most countries including those in the developing world have formal training programs, most which include written curricula.** Twenty-nine of the 30 residents interviewed stated that there was a formal training program, which they were meant to follow. The exception was an African surgeon, who stated, *"From six weeks into the job, I had no regular supervision. I once was on-call for 30 days at a stretch at a peripheral hospital. I'm essentially self-taught and I've been in independent practice almost from the beginning of my residency."*

Although most training schemes have agreed curricula many programs do not follow their own curricula. Five of the 29 surgeons said although they did have a formal curriculum it had little significance for them. This was well expressed by two trainees from Europe, *"Cases come in every day and you have to deal with them. It's the cases that dictate what you learn. We have the occasional lecture, but I just don't feel like we are adhering to a formal syllabus even though we have one."*

All but one of the trainees questioned had to pass final examinations and accessing education to pass these exams was a powerful educational driver for many. The exception is Scandinavia where a complex 360-degree continuous assessment process takes the place of a final exam. In addition to the final exams, half of the residents had intermediate exams. Passing these exams is necessary to progress to the remainder of the training program.

The length of the residency program varies considerably around the world. The shortest is in India, where the formal program lasts for 3 years. The longest is in Great Britain, where the program lasts between 5 or 6 years. **Those trainees who have a very short residency period tend not to go into independent practice at the end of their residency, but continue working in the hospitals in which they were residents for a further period of time, usually under supervision.** This career pathway is commonest in India.

All the trainees interviewed were in a training program in both orthopedics and traumatology. None of the trainees were training in general surgery. The general surgical route into trauma surgery is now very rare, being only found in the Netherlands, Austria, and Switzerland. Germany has recently changed its training programs to train future orthopedic trauma surgeons as orthopedic and not general surgeons.

Residency should be supervised but the degree of supervision varies greatly from scheme to scheme and country to country. *"We have very good supervision of our operative surgery. We all have to fill in log books so if the supervising body picks up that we are doing too much independent surgery then the training scheme itself is at risk."*

"You get to know which consultant will come in to help you and which will prefer you get on with surgery on your own. They would always come in if you really asked but we are not encouraged to do so. I find that the senior nurses are really helpful when you get stuck."

The hours worked by residents also varies considerably from the 48-hour maximum being introduced within the European Union to the 108-hour weeks that characterized residency in earlier times. These changes have met with variable reactions from trainees many of which were negative. *"Having to work a 48 hour week is a real pain because it means that we will have to work shifts for the first 2 years. This makes continuity of care difficult. It also means that we miss out on some teaching sessions."*

The reduction in working time is felt by some to reflect the new life-work balance needs of today's residents. No resident interviewed in this study expressed this view.

3.1   Today's residents: learning needs and preferences

Experience of interviewees

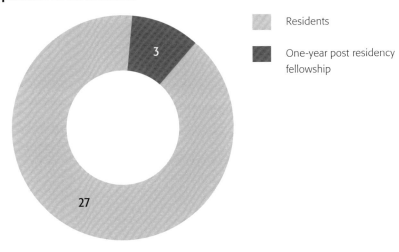

Residents

One-year post residency fellowship

Thirty surgeons in training were interviewed in this part of the study. Twenty-seven of these were still in residency and three were partway through a one-year post residency fellowship. None of the surgeons in training had passed their final exams or were board certified.

Origin of interviewees

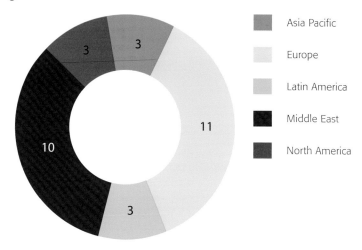

- Asia Pacific
- Europe
- Latin America
- Middle East
- North America

Eleven of the residents came from Europe, three from Latin America, three from the Middle East, ten from North America, and three from Asia Pacific.

3.1.1   Characteristic forms of learning

There was remarkable consistency when current residents were asked about their typical learning experiences. **Twenty-two of the 30 trainees stated that the typical way they learnt was by gaining experience on the job.** Ideally they would see a patient either in the emergency room or the clinic and work the patient up. To do this they would get help from a variety of educational resources. They would then proceed to treat the patient, ideally under supervision, and continue on to follow up the patient. *"Residency is still a form of apprenticeship. The way you really learn is to first see a patient in the emergency room or clinic and then formulate a treatment program, carry it out, and then follow the patient up. We have a lot of formal teaching on our program but what sticks is the clinical experience."* Other typical learning experiences include one surgeon who said that his typical learning was through the Internet. *"The usual way I learn is to use the Internet. I see a problem and go straight online. I usually use Wheeless to start with and then may go into PubMed if I have time. I like the fact that I can access the information when I need it."* Another two felt that their typical learning was in preparing themselves for examination. One said his typical learning was by working through a formal curriculum, and two said their typical way of learning was by being mentored by a senior figure. It should be noted that both of these mentored trainees were undergoing fellowship training.

3.1.2   Best learning

There was less uniformity when residents were asked to describe their best learning experiences but **14 of the 30 residents interviewed felt that their best learning experiences occurred while learning on the job.**
"I saw this man in the ER with a fractured forearm. It was technically an open fracture so we had to get on with it. My senior resident wasn't well and so I called in the attending. I spend about an hour reviewing the anatomy and he then took me through the case. I will never forget how he taught me to dissect and to use the anatomy to my advantage. That experience completely changed the way I perform surgery."

Four of the trainees felt that their best learning experience was learning on the Internet. One of these residents accessed regular eLearning modules, which were made available to him by his local training association. *"Every month we get a new eLearning module. That way whatever is going on in our hospital we are sure that we will cover the complete syllabus necessary to pass the exams. It's a perfect way to learn because I can do it at a time to suit me."* The other three used the Internet for communication and information gathering. One surgeon had become part of a learning community set up online. *"Under the direction of my boss we have set up an online closed group from several different hospitals to discuss clinical problems. We contact each other on a regular basis and it works best when my boss moderates the sessions. It's great because we get to discuss each other's problems."*

Four trainees commented that their best learning experience was attending hospital meetings. All four agreed that the reason was two-fold. Firstly, they had to prepare themselves for these meetings and that was a stimulus for their learning. Secondly, they all agreed that the discussion and feedback that occurred at these meetings was very important for their learning. *"Although preparing for teaching sessions is hard, it gives you the stimulus to go and look things up. It is amazing what you can find. When it comes to the meeting itself the best bit is to hear different opinions. When the bosses disagree then it gets really interesting."* All four were talking about clinical meetings held on a regular basis within the hospitals. Journal clubs were mentioned as good learning experiences by six of the trainees. They commented that preparation and interaction were important, but four of the trainees stated that there was a further element in these, *"Being a resident in my country is a very competitive business. Attending the journal clubs and showing off your knowledge is a very good way to ensure that your bosses know that you are doing a good job."* One surgeon identified being with a mentor as his best learning experience, two surgeons identified going on the AO Principle Course as being their best learning experience, one surgeon felt that reading books was his best learning experience, and one surgeon said that he could not identify what method of learning was best for him in his residency.

3.1.3   People

Twenty of the 30 trainees felt that interacting with people in their hospitals is a very important part of their learning. The most important interactions occurred with senior colleagues, attendings, and consultants. However, ten trainees mentioned that interaction with senior residents was often critical for them. *"You can look things up online or use a book. But nothing compares with the ability to discuss cases. I often take my case to three or four attendings to get as many viewpoints as I can. Talking with the bosses is the best way to learn."* Six of the 30 commented that their seniors were often not present and that they were largely self-taught. These trainees were widely distributed in their countries of origin, but none were in North America. *"If a case is scheduled for the morning then it is very likely one of the bosses will give you a hand. In the afternoon they go off to their own practices and the major source of help is the senior residents. In the evening and night time you are on your own."*

3.1.4   Books

Books are the most popular way of accessing information and remarkably were rated by many as being more important than the Internet. All trainees but one bought standard textbooks at the start of their training, the exception being a surgeon from Africa who could not afford to buy any textbooks. Books were characteristically read on a subject basis at the beginning of training, but the use of books declined during residency and books were increasingly used to answer more specific clinical questions. *"When I arrived at my hospital I was told to buy three books—Campbells, Rockwood and Green, and Hoppenfeld. To start with I read them every evening, chapter by chapter but soon I was only reading what was relevant to next day's cases. As time went on I used books less and less but they are still important for exams and preparing to do unusual cases."* Seven of the trainees commented that books were an important part of the training syllabus and reading standard textbooks was important for preparing for examinations. Campbell's was by far the most important textbook for all those trainees interviewed who had access to it. *"Campbells is the Bible. Our weekly meetings are based around the book. It's got all the references you will ever need."* Two trainees felt that books were out of date and preferred accessing information online. *"Books are expensive and easily out-of-date. No navigation is possible. The standard texts are not well written. I much prefer to access information online."*

Surgeons' preferences as to the format used by books—electronic or print—is variable and changing. Some surgeons prefer a printed version particularly if they needed to study individual diagrams. Others much prefer an electronic version. *"I would much rather have an electronic book. Online access to information is by far the most important thing. I have access to an online textbook with electronic updates."*

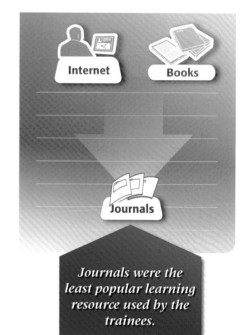

Journals were the least popular learning resource used by the trainees.

3.1.5   Journals

Journals are the least popular learning resource used by the trainees. Two surgeons had great difficulty in accessing journals. For some, journals became more important towards the end of training. In the UK critical analysis of a journal article was part of the final examination. *"Campbell's is the syllabus. I don't use journals yet, but will have to do so for the final exams. As part of our finals we have to critically review a paper—statistics and all."*

Of those trainees who did read journals, all of them used electronic access. Four trainees had training programs which gave them free online access to journals through their medical libraries.

The commonest reason for accessing journals was preparation for clinical meetings. *"We have clinical meetings every week during term time based around defined topics. Four times a year you have to present at these meetings. You are assigned a boss to work with you and if you are lucky he may give you some key references. If not you use the Internet to find some up-to-date articles. I use Google as my search engine. It gets me there in the end but most of the stuff on the first page is commercial."*

When journals were used to prepare for clinical meetings access was always online via a search engine, of which PubMed or Google were by far the commonest used. Only four of the 30 trainees actually read journals as they came out to keep themselves up-to-date. All four of these trainees were from developing countries.

3.1.6   Internet

Twenty-nine of the 30 trainees used the Internet on a daily basis. The exception did not have access to the Internet. All trainees used the Internet as a communication tool and 26 of the trainees used electronic log-books to store their own information.

All the trainees used the Internet to get information. The commonest indication was to prepare themselves for presentations and meetings within the hospital.

The second commonest indication was to investigate a case they were dealing with. It should be noted, however, that the majority of trainees prefer to seek interaction with peers and seniors when faced with clinical issues. *"If you have got 10 minutes or so to work up a case just before the morning trauma round then I always go online and use Wheeless. When the round starts, however, it is the discussion with the chiefs that helps me best. It's the only way you get to ask questions and we are lucky because our chiefs encourage us to ask."*

Four of the trainees stated that access to the Internet was their best learning experience. One trainee liked eLearning but stated that there were a very few good eLearning sites available. Two surgeons were members of online communities, where case forums existed and discussion and interactivity occurred. One website had been set up by the local trainees in the Middle East. The second was sponsored by a training organization in Latin America. *"Our boss is very keen on using the Internet. He has set up an Internet club of trainees. We meet online most weeks and discuss cases. He is usually there to moderate. We can present our own cases, which we post online in advance. It really works well and we can involve all of our trainees who work in different hospitals."*

The AO Surgery Reference and Traumaline—an award winning Internet-based information resource published by this study's sponsor—were accessed by half of the trainees. Those that did access the site felt that it was very useful, but six trainees commented that they felt that it should be organized along procedural lines rather than along the lines of treating a particular pathology.

One residency program provided online PDFs and lectures. Four of the trainees commented that they liked watching treatment-related videos on the Internet. **Nineteen of the residents used Wheeless electronic book.** They liked the fact that they could access information rapidly. They also liked the fact that Wheeless dealt with orthopedics as well as traumatology.

The most powerful advocate for eLearning stated, *"There is a conflict between service and training. I am a member of an online community and we interact around the cases. The AO should form its own online community. The AO should develop simulators and more eLearning."*

At the end of the interviews the residents were asked what single thing could be done for them by an educational organization that would improve the care that they were able to give to their patients. **Although the Internet had not featured as the most valued learning modality for most of the residents interviewed, improvements to online accessible education dominated responses about what they would like in the future.**

Fifteen interviewees from all career stages made a request for new and/or improved online services relating to education. Eleven of these 15 surgeons were residents-in-training and only four came from surgeons who were in independent practice.

It is clear from this data that online services are highly valued by residents-in-training and there is a clear implication that the existing online resources are inadequate.

Criticisms that were made related to many different aspects of online education. One resident said, *"There is no shortage of information for me on the net. What I would like is for someone to develop an online search engine that takes me where I need to go. Whichever search engine I use at present, it always gives me too much information and even PubMed often does not give me what I need."* Another resident stated, *"There is nothing out there with eLearning. I think we should have eLearning with MCQ self-assessments. It is clearly the future for medical education because education can be done at any time to fit in with a busy schedule."*

It must be noted, however, that that individual was currently preparing a PhD thesis on online learning. Perhaps much of the feelings expressed by residents could be summed up by a third resident, who stated, *"Really, I want you to provide me instant access to relevant information at the touch of a button. I want to be able to use my iPhone as I go to the OR and find the part of the operation I am about to do that I am unclear about explained in a clear manner. I would like an app."*

3.1.7   Courses

All the trainees interviewed had attended the **AO Principles Course. All but one of them rated the course as being a very positive educational experience.** *"Taking the AO Principles Course was the best educational experience I had at the start of my residency. I had been doing some trauma cases before I got accepted into the program. The course taught me the reasons why I had been doing what I had. It also showed me that there was a better way of looking at some problems. I used to think of the fracture. The course taught me to think of the patient."*

Two aspects of the course attracted the most positive comments. These were the practicals and the discussions. *"The best parts of the course were the practicals. I had been hanging onto retractors for six months so it was the first time I got to use the instruments themselves. I also found that the practicals let me understand things I had not understood from the lectures."*

The practicals were felt to be important by all, but four of the trainees stressed that the practicals were designed for surgeons in the very early stages of their careers and were much less valuable if the trainee was experienced. *"Because there was a waiting list for the course in my country I did not do the course until I had almost finished my residency. By that time I was doing a lot of trauma surgery independently. The practicals were not that much use to me."*

Those trainees who had taken the course at a later stage of their residency liked the fact that the clinical issues were discussed in a variety of teaching formats including discussion. *"I liked the case discussions. It gave me a chance to ask about the clinical problems I had been facing. Many of the cases we looked at were too basic for me but we did get some good discussion going."*

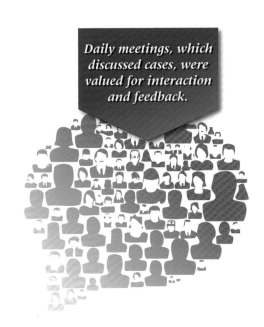

Daily meetings, which discussed cases, were valued for interaction and feedback.

3.1.8   Hospital meetings

Meetings within the hospital seemed to be very important to trainees. Twenty-seven of 30 trainees had regular meetings. Daily meetings, which discussed cases, were valued for the interactiion and the feedback that was given. More formal training meetings and journal clubs were valued because of the interaction and the incentive that they give to learn because the participants had to prepare for the sessions.

3.1.9   Mentoring

Mentoring occurred very rarely during residency, which is a surprising finding given the fact that many training programs now claim mentoring to be a major element in their programs. Only three of the 30 candidates mentioned mentoring as important element in their learning, two of which were taking fellowships.

3.2 Today's residents: educational needs and implications for teaching organizations

- **Teaching and learning in the field of orthopedic traumatology is now almost universally part of a residency training program in orthopedics.** Although trauma may represent up to 80% of the operative workload of a surgeon-in-training, teaching about trauma only represents between 25% and 40% of the training program syllabus.

- The current success enjoyed by the online "Wheeles' Textbook of Orthopaedics" is due to the broad scope of the content. It is largely used by residents who want instant access to a minimal information data set used most often in the context of a daily trauma round. Educational organizations should be aware that this service is important to residents when they are preparing for clinical meetings. Residents do not want comprehensive information at that time. **Incorporating navigation into existing standard texts may provide such a resource that could be accessed on a hand held device.**

- **All residents in training have to pass examinations or other forms of assessment. Preparation for examinations is a huge driver for residents to seek education.** Currently, books and review articles accessed through the Internet form the basis of this preparation. The teaching organization might consider developing online-based resources specifically targeted at passing the examinations utilizing existing educational resources.

- Hospital meetings occur in nearly every residency program and are considered to be very important by most of the residents interviewed. **For the day-to-day trauma round type of meeting, Internet-based education is ideal.** The use of the AO Surgery Reference was common amongst those who were interviewed. Although most were happy with the service, several commented that they would prefer the organization of the portal to be based on surgical procedures rather than on pathology.

- More formal training meetings, including journal clubs, are also rated as being important. Currently, residents access information for these meetings through the Internet using search engines of which PubMed and Google are the commonest.

- Residency teaching is now much more organized than in the past with most training schemes having an agreed curriculum. Formal teaching sessions occur on a regular basis for most residents. Despite this most residents feel that most of their best learning occurs when they encounter a case, work it up and then follow it through. Although part of that work-up may be through an Internet-based educational tool, most of the residents stated clearly that interaction, either with their peers or attendings, was the most important element in a successful learning experience. **Teaching organizations should consider training surgeons to become more effective teachers in the workplace as part of their faculty development programs.** The teaching skills required for successful education of course participants overlap greatly with those required for successful informal work place teaching and learning.

- **The AO Principle Course was very highly valued by nearly every resident interviewed.** Other courses attended by residents are not so highly valued except those that feature a significant amount of practical exercises. For example, cadaveric workshops to study anatomy and arthroscopic workshops to study arthroscopy. Residents state clearly that the Principles Course is a central part of their education.

  Residents are clear that this course should be taken very early in surgical training which is now the case in most countries. Historically some senior surgeons took the Principles Course late in their surgical career. This was because of the lack of availability of education in their countries when they were residents. Some countries are still at a very early stage of their development and in these countries consideration should be given to modifying some elements of the practicals and discussions to reflect the seniority of the course participants.

  The practicals are the most highly valued of all the teaching modalities although the combination of lecture, discussion, and practical in the form of blended learning is also widely appreciated particularly by those surgeons who took the course very late in their residency. **Interactivity and practicals are the jewels in the AO Principles Course crown. Although significant elements of the course could be made available online, the key elements of the practicals and the small group discussions cannot.** Cost and time are elements that do affect surgeons-in-training but the majority of residents like the idea of getting away from the work environment for a clearly defined study period. The vast majority of surgeons attending these courses are sponsored either by an implant manufacturer or their teaching institution.

- Journals are not rated as being very important in the sense that few people now access journals and read them on a regular basis. However, journal articles remain very important in terms of an educational resource. This results in a dilemma for potential publishers of journals. **The demand for material included in journals remains great but the desire of an individual surgeon to purchase the journal is lacking.** Material available in journals is now accessed via the Internet using a search engine and many residents read and quote the available abstract rather read the article as a whole. Current common practice is for teaching institutions to purchase access to journal articles on behalf of their trainees and marketing of journals, especially new ones will have to be innovative and reflect current practice.

3.3   How has residency changed over time?

3.3.1   Residency as remembered by surgeons starting independent practice

Origin of interviewees

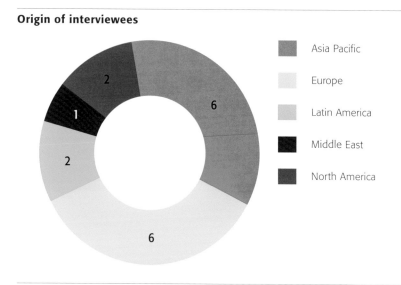

Asia Pacific

Europe

Latin America

Middle East

North America

Sixteen surgeons who were just starting independent practice were interviewed for this part of the study. All were within 5 years of completing a residency program. Six surgeons were from Europe, two from North America, six from Asia Pacific, two from Latin America, and one from the Middle East.

The message given by those surgeons who left residency programs up to 5 years ago is that residency in their time was similar in many ways to the way it is today. Their belief that most learning occurred from treating patients on the job was identical to the feelings of today's residents.

There were however some differences. Although curricula had been introduced their use was less than it is today. Interaction with people in the work place was very important but the degree of direct supervision from seniors was less. Books were the next best learning resource with many surgeons having problems with Internet access, particularly in the developing world.

Ten of the 16 surgeons interviewed felt that 5 years ago residency typically consisted of learning on the job. Although three quarters of the surgeons said there was a form of curriculum, most stated that the reality of their learning was dictated by the cases that came into the hospital. Only two surgeons felt that formal teaching within their program was the typical way in which they learned. Two surgeons felt that reading books was the way they usually learned and two surgeons felt that typical learning was achieved through discussion with peers and seniors.

Nine surgeons felt that their best learning occurred as a result of experience gained by treating patients. *"Hands on surgery was the best. I learned by operating on patients."* Six surgeons felt that their best learning occurred as result of meetings held in their hospitals. Two types of meeting were identified. The first were clinical meetings typically held at the start of the day to discuss the cases to be operated on that day and what had occurred during the previous 24 hours. These meetings were valued because of the discussion that took place and because feedback was instantly available. A surgeon from India identified another element in these meetings, *"I had to be seen to be better than the other residents and hospital meetings were my opportunity to do so. I would prepare my cases very carefully using my books and try to make a good impression."* One surgeon felt that the mentoring relationship he enjoyed with his professor was the most important element in his learning while a resident.

The relationship between the surgeons and their chiefs during residency was very variable. Only one of the surgeons interviewed identified a close mentor-type relationship with his professor. Six of the 17 stated that being taken through a case by their professor was the best learning experience of their residency. Four of the surgeons felt that they were essentially self-taught and were often left alone at night having to operate on their own. *"You got to know which of the chiefs came in the evening and which did not. In a real emergency there was never a problem in getting some help but some bosses expected more than others in terms of how much you did on your own."*

Books were a popular learning resource. Surgeons commented that books were very helpful for examinations. Nearly everybody interviewed bought standard textbooks when starting their residency. As nowadays there was a general tendency to use books less as residency proceeded. Surgeons used books in different ways, as they got more experienced. Initially they read the book or relevant chapter as a whole. Later in their residency they used books only if they had a specific case-based problem or if they were preparing for an examination.

Journals were used infrequently and then usually towards the end of training. The most common use for journals was to prepare for teaching meetings but one surgeon who trained in the former Soviet block commented, *"My best experiences were being alone at night and having to operate on my own. All I had were some old Russian textbooks. I found that the Journal of Bone and Joint Surgery was my best resource."*

Six of the 17 surgeons did not use the Internet on a regular basis when they were residents due to the fact that they did not have access to the Internet at that time. **All of the surgeons who did have access to the Internet used it for communications and for information gathering.** PubMed and Google were the major search engines used. Three surgeons commented that their use of the Internet was markedly hampered by their lack of skills in speaking English. Very little research information is available online outside the English language and there is a perception that the quality of articles published in some native languages is not as good as in the major journals. *"Getting access to the Internet was not easy. We only had a single computer connected to the Internet and it was very slow by comparison with now. Many times you just gave up and went off to the library to look it up in a book. All that has now changed."*

No surgeon reported using the Internet for eLearning. The commonest reason for Internet use was to prepare for clinical meetings and information was accessed through a search engine.

Four of the 17 surgeons did not have access to formal educational courses such as the AO Principles Course during their residency. Those surgeons who did take such courses were very positive about their learning experiences and expressed identical views to today's residents about their feelings.

Hospital meetings were an extremely important part of learning in residency for this group of surgeons. They rated meetings as being important because they gave the opportunity to discuss things. One surgeon commented, *"The patient review meetings were open and interactive. It was the best time to find out how you were getting along."*

Formal mentoring was very unusual in this group of surgeons, and although one surgeon formed a close mentoring relationship with his senior trainer, no formal mentoring processes were identified as being part of any surgeon's residency.

3.3.2   Residency as remembered by surgeons now acquiring specialization skills

Origin of interviewees

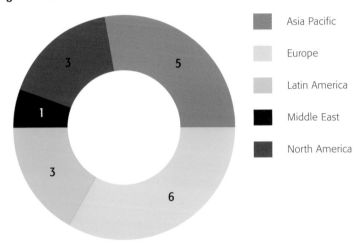

Asia Pacific

Europe

Latin America

Middle East

North America

Eighteen surgeons who are currently acquiring expertise were interviewed for this part of the study. Five surgeons were from Asia Pacific, six from Europe, three from North America, three surgeons from Latin America, and one surgeon was from the Middle East. The surgeons who were interviewed were between 5 and 10 years from the completion of residency. Two of the 18 surgeons interviewed continue to work under a degree of supervision at their places of residency. They had a degree of independent practice but still had to refer their decisions to the head of the department.

Ten to fifteen years ago residency was very different from what is experienced today. Formal curricula were less common and some programs did not have formal end of residency examinations. Books were more important as reference sources than now and journals were the best way of keeping up to date. For many surgeons, however, especially those in the developing world, getting access to journals was a big problem. Internet access was rare and the full potential of the Internet was not yet appreciated. The level of supervision enjoyed by residents was significantly less than today although some surgeons reported close and supportive relationships with their seniors. Interaction with people inside the hospital, especially senior residents, was important.

Despite these differences the surgeons who were interviewed shared the belief, held by all generations of surgeons interviewed, that **in essence residency consisted of learning through on-the-job experience.**

Fourteen of the 18 surgeons interviewed stated that their residency training was dictated by the cases that came into the hospital during their residency. The classic pattern of learning was: see a patient, make a diagnosis, do the operation, and follow it up.

Ten of the 17 surgeons said that their best learning experiences were self-taught. *"The best learning occurred when you were on your own at night. You never knew what would come in and you just had to do your best using books and getting advice from other staff. Having to do something is a powerful way to learn."*

In stark contrast, five of the surgeons identified a mentoring figure as being their best learning resource during their residency. These relationships were never formalized but were in practice a true mentoring relationship. *"From the first day I arrived in the hospital I became aware that X was the dominant figure. He seemed to care about each of his residents and I used his help and advice long after I left my teaching hospital."*

The relationship between the residents and their seniors was very varied. Some comments were not positive, *"Professors were remote." "The lectures given by professors were no good. I had largely independent practice from a very early stage." "I was nearly always unsupervised. I was thrown in at the deep end. I was self-taught."*

Books were a very important learning resource for this group of surgeons. All surgeons but one rated books as being very important. The one surgeon who disagreed had great difficulty in accessing textbooks during his residency. Problems with access to material were an even greater influence when the role of journals was discussed. Journals were used for examination purposes and for preparing for clinical meetings but were very difficult to access in the developing world and in the former Soviet block.

Twelve of the 18 surgeons did not have access to the Internet when they were in residency. Those that did used it significantly less than current surgeons, mainly because of difficulty in accessing information due to slow or intermittent connections. When used, the dominant search engines were PubMed and Google.

Eight of the 18 surgeons did not have access to educational courses such as the AO Principles Course during their residency. Those that did have access to such courses rated them significantly less in terms of its value than the younger surgeons who were interviewed. This was mainly due to the fact that many surgeons took the course too late. *"By the time I did the AO Principles Course, I had such extensive experience that the course was largely a waste of time for me. When I did the Advanced Course, I enjoyed the discussions."*

Meetings were important to this group of surgeons while they were in residency training, but slightly less so than those who are currently in residency training. *"Although we were meant to have regular teaching meetings on a Friday afternoon, attendance from the chiefs was usually very poor. After a while it became quite normal to plan to miss the meeting if you could."*

Preparation for meetings was again thought to be one of the reasons that meetings were valued as a useful learning tool. Interaction was also highly valued.

Five of the 18 surgeons said they enjoyed a mentoring-type relationship with their senior trainer, which is a surprisingly large number. All these relationships, however, were personal ones rather than formal mentoring relationships set up in the context of the training program.

3.3.3   Residency as remembered by expert surgeons

Origin of interviewees

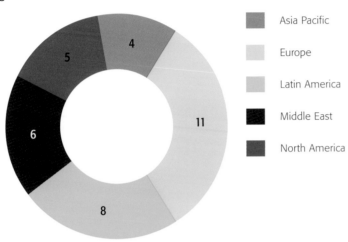

Legend:
- Asia Pacific
- Europe
- Latin America
- Middle East
- North America

Thirty-five established experts in trauma surgery were interviewed. Eight surgeons were from Latin America, eleven were from Europe, five were from North America, six were from the Middle East, and four were from Asia Pacific.

The surgeons interviewed varied considerably in their level of experience—ranging between 10 and 30 years from the completion of their residency. Their memories therefore relate to sub-specialty training between 1985 and 2000.

Twenty or more years ago residency was totally different to that experienced by today's residents. Formal curricula were rare, and if they did exist, were often not followed. Most surgeons interviewed felt that they had been largely self-taught, relying on experience gained on the job, helped by books. Twenty-nine of the 36 surgeons stated they were either self-taught or learned on the job. *"I did not really have much teaching. The best teaching occurred when a consultant took me through humeral plating. Consultants always said to me—if you have a problem just call me. You never did."*

The relationship between residents and their trainers was variable. Over half of the surgeons interviewed commented that their bosses were either not there or difficult to contact. Most teaching given by seniors was done in the context of meetings, which were thought to be very important. One surgeon commented, *"The professors were there before noon, senior residents were there in the afternoon, and in the evening, and you just had to get on with it yourself."*

Perhaps, not surprisingly, books were the most important learning resource for this group of surgeons. These surgeons did not have Internet access during their resident training. They often did not have a formal curriculum. Most of them had limited or no supervision by seniors. Standard textbooks were therefore critical to their learning, although three had difficulty in accessing even these. *"All we had were some old books in the library. They were very out of date but they were all we had. I learned how to reduce fractures and put them in plaster from Charnleys book, which was then 20 years old. I still think it is a good book and I would recommend it to my residents."*

Journals were surprisingly important to many of the surgeons interviewed. Even though many of them had difficulty in accessing journals, most tried to get hold of journals when they could and then read them cover-to-cover. *"It was always a good day when the latest copy of the JBJS arrived in the post. It was an opportunity to find out what was new. I would start by reading the articles I thought were most interesting and go on from there. I even read the letters to the editor."*

It is tempting to speculate that the increased use of journals and the switch from case-based reading to general reading was due to the fact that none of the surgeons interviewed had access to the Internet while they were a resident.

Thirteen of the 36 surgeons did not have access to formal educational courses such as the AO Principle Course during their residency. This reflects the lack of widespread AO Education at that time. Those who attended AO courses thought that they were very important but felt that it should be taken early in training. This opinion resonates with data from the other groups interviewed. Practical skill training was again the most highly rated of the teaching modalities, but interactivity was also thought to be very important.

Hospital meetings, when present, were very highly rated. The time and effort required to prepare for the meetings were thought to be the best drivers of learning. Large numbers of surgeons, however, did not have any hospital meetings.

Only one of the surgeons interviewed felt that they had a mentoring-type relationship with a senior surgeon. The concept of mentoring was not really present in residency training in those days and most surgeons interviewed felt that residency was an apprenticeship based on working out the solution to your patient's problems largely on your own.

3.4   Resident training: implications for a teaching organization

The surgeons who were interviewed describe marked changes that have occurred in residency training over the last 25 years. All generations of surgeons agree that many aspects of an apprenticeship—learning on the job—have been and will remain the most important part of training. However, there have clearly been a series of changes, which in turn have impacted the way the most effective teaching and learning occurs during residency training.

- **Formal curricula have been developed together with an examination system built around the curriculum.**

This has led to an increased need to access information across the whole spectrum of trauma and orthopedics. Historically it was possible to learn merely by experience. Nowadays residents are expected to know what to do even if they have not encountered the clinical problem. This need for information is being met by an increased use of the Internet. Internet usage is however plagued by a difficulty in accessing information that is relevant and a lack of clarity about what available information is valid and what is not. *"If you Google "distal radial fractures" you will find over 170,000 links. On the first page there are twelfe sites that are blatantly commercial and Wikipedia. There is no way of knowing what is good so you tend to rely on those sites you feel you can trust like the American Academy of Orthopedic Surgeons."*

Teaching organizations need to focus not only on providing information but also helping residents access relevant, valid, and significant information from the vast amount available online and from other channels.

- **Supervision of surgical procedures by senior staff is much more common.**

Increased supervision is clearly a good thing both for trainees and patients alike. Genuine supervision as opposed to doing the case and letting the trainee watch is time consuming and requires teaching skills on the part of the trainer, which he or she may not have been exposed to as a trainee. Being an effective teacher of practical skills is therefore more important than ever, especially when the reduction in trainee working hours is decreasing rapidly. *"X is a really good teacher. He won't let you do the case until you have discussed it with him and he is sure you know what you are going to do. Afterwards I get really good feedback. X is not typical. Y won't let you do anything. He starts off by assisting but as soon as any problems occur he takes over and that's it."*

Teaching organizations should consider including the teaching of practical skills in the workplace as part of their faculty training programs. This would help prepare faculty for teaching practical skills on educational courses.

- **Internet usage is increasing but current trainees find existing learning resources inadequate.**

The Internet is now the major reference tool of residents. They use the Internet for a variety of tasks including social networking sites. **The development of apps using small hand held devices has opened up the possibility of accessing information at any time and in any place.** Selection of material remains a problem. Although many residents raise the issue of eLearning as an adjunct to their studies, most still value the interactivity obtained from contact with people, either informally on the job or in clinical meetings. *"When I go to the OR to do a case I know what I want to do. I know what implant I am going to use. I know what technique I will use. I don't know how to strip the supinator of the bone safely without endangering the posterior interosseous nerve. So what I want is to use my iPhone and use an app which tells me this and nothing else."*

Teaching organizations need to consider adapting their current educational material to make it navigable and available online through small hand held devices.

There appears to be very little effective eLearning occurring during residency. Teaching organizations need to explore why this is the case and what needs to be done.

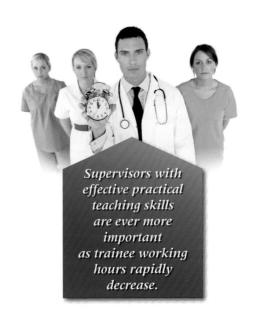

Supervisors with effective practical teaching skills are ever more important as trainee working hours rapidly decrease.

4 Beginning of practice

Chapter 4
Beginning of practice

Starting surgical practice can be the most stressful stage in a surgeon's career. Interaction with colleagues and informal mentorships are highlighted as the primary mode of learning at this career stage. Interestingly, interviews reveal that current educational resources do not seem to meet the needs of the majority.

The beginning of practice stage marks the period of time in a surgeon's career immediately after completing his or her residency/fellowship. **Of all the career stages examined, it is the most variable.**

Origin of interviewees

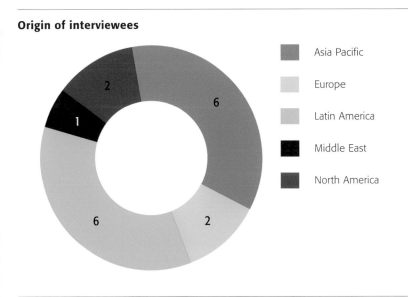

Asia Pacific

Europe

Latin America

Middle East

North America

Of the seventeen surgeons interviewed who were within 5 years of the completion of residency, six were from Asia Pacific, two were from North America, six were from Europe, one was from Middle East, and two were from Latin America.

4.1   Career patterns

Two distinct career patterns were clear. **Nine of the 17 surgeons interviewed continued to work under a degree of supervision** often at their places of residency. They were given a degree of independent practice from the start but in general terms had to refer most decisions to a senior professor. The majority of these had undergone a relatively short period of residency training. These surgeons were most commonly found in Europe and in Asia Pacific. **Generally speaking, these surgeons found the transition to the beginning of practice easier than those surgeons who went straight into independent practice.** They relied heavily on support networks within their institutions. That support network consisted of their professor and peers.

"After I got my MS I became an associate professor in my teaching hospital. I had to teach and supervise the residents but the professor continued to control most of my work. I had a degree of independent practice but all the key decisions were made by the professor. It was a gradual process of getting more and more independence but the Prof was always there when I was in doubt. After another 3 years I was made an assistant professor and really started to have my own patients."

The second group of surgeons contained those who moved straight from residency/fellowship into true independent practice. **These surgeons found the change into independent practice was a relatively stressful experience.** *"This was a very, very difficult transition for me. To start with, I was very reliant on my friends and my seniors. I frequently did not know what to do." "This was very hard to start with. We had weekly meetings that are good for discussion but I was very reliant on my colleagues for help and advice."*

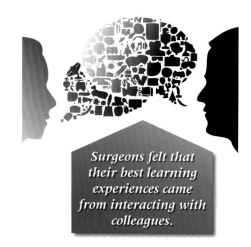

Surgeons felt that their best learning experiences came from interacting with colleagues.

4.2   Beginning of practice: learning needs and preferences

4.2.1   Characteristic forms of learning
The overwhelming majority of surgeons (ten of the 17 surgeons,) said that they were largely self-taught. *"Arriving at my new hospital I found that I was on call the following night. A talar dislocation came in—something which I had never seen in my residency. There was no one to ask for help so I got out the books and did the case. It went well. You just have to get on with it but know your limitations."*

Five felt that their typical form of learning was a mentoring experience with a senior colleague.

"After my fellowship I realized that I could not develop a pelvis and acetabular service on my own. So every month I collected my X-rays together and drove to my old teachers hospital to show him what I had done and discuss what needed to be done with the new patients. He was genuinely interested in me as a person and we began a friendship that I am sure will last."

One commented that his typical form of teaching and learning was accessing the Internet.

4.2.2   Best learning experiences

Best learning was markedly different from typical learning. **Ten of the 17 surgeons interviewed felt that their best learning experience was interacting with mentors, senior colleagues, and peers.** *"I felt very isolated. Although I was helped by a fellowship, most of the help came from a senior professor who would always come in on request." "I kept in touch with my old chief and whenever I came across a problem I would call him up and he would be happy to discuss the case. He made me realize that I had to adapt my practice to the situation I found myself in and not just do what the books said I should."*

Of the remaining surgeons two felt that their best learning experience was being self-taught. One felt attending a principles level course was his best learning experience. Two felt that the Internet was their best learning experience. *"When you are on your own and have responsibility for the patient having access to a step-by-step online guide to patient treatment is fantastic."*

One surgeon commented that his best learning experience came from having to achieve publications. *"Having to achieve publications meant that I had to look things up. Review articles were best. I read journals to give me the edge over other people at my stage. I am very competitive."*

Another surgeon had developed an online learning community with surgeons at the same stage in their careers. The community focused on providing help to pass examinations and teach ATLS.

4.2.3   People

Ten of the 17 surgeons interviewed stated that interaction with people was by far the most important and best learning experience they had during this stage in their career. Although the majority of interactions were with people who worked in the same institution, three of the surgeons interviewed relied on contacts from their previous employment in senior residency or fellowships.

Of all the surgeon's career stages examined by this study, the beginning of practice is the one where surgeons are most reliant on interpersonal relationships and it is the only stage of the career path where a mentoring type relationship features so significantly in the lives of many surgeons. Yet none of the surgeons questioned had a formal system of mentorship within their hospitals. The mentorship process was based on a personal one-on-one relationship and it is interesting to note that two of these relationships began as a result of fellowships.

4.2.4   Books

Although books remain a useful learning tool for many surgeons beginning their practice, far fewer of them identify books as being an important source of education compared with surgeons who are still in training. When books are used, it is usually on a case basis rather than reading a section or chapter.

4.2.5   Journals

Although the use of journals is more popular with surgeons at the beginning of their practice than that it is with residents, most surgeons do not think reading journals is an important part of their learning. When surgeons do access journals the majority access journal articles via an Internet search engine. Two surgeons interviewed still subscribe to journals and read them on a monthly basis but the majority of surgeon's only access journal articles when they are clinically indicated. *"Really, it's a slow switch from books to journals. Initially, you browse and then increasingly your reading becomes case-based. It's like learning to ride a bike."*

4.2.6   Internet

All surgeons but one use the Internet. All Internet users use it for communication and for accessing information, usually via one of three search engines: Google, PubMed, and OVID. One surgeon did not have access to the Internet. The most innovative use of the Internet was that of the surgeon who had set up a learning community. *"Hospitals in my country are often many kilometers from each other. We all get together at national meetings but otherwise units are isolated from each other. I decided to set up a web-based club for interested surgeons. We meet up every week and the discussion is around cases that get posted online. We tend to spend some time on a particular type of fracture and then move on to other problem areas. There is always an acetabulum to look at."* None of the surgeons reported that they use the Internet for eLearning and the AO website, PubMed, Ovid, and Google were the only specific sites that were named apart from the Wheeless electronic textbook.

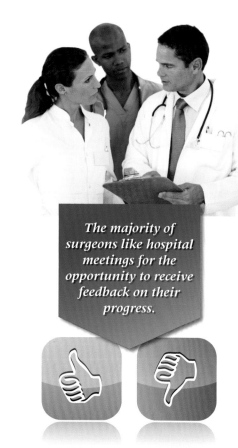

The majority of surgeons like hospital meetings for the opportunity to receive feedback on their progress.

4.2.7   Courses

Formal educational courses are less important to surgeons in the beginning of practice than in residency. Those surgeons who took a principles level course during this stage in their careers were less enthusiastic about the course than the residents. The majority of them commented that they had taken the course too late in their career and they felt that the course was best targeted to surgeons in an early stage of their practice. *"I now teach on the Principles Course and I think it is great for my residents. I did the course when I had been in independent practice for 2 years. Some bits of it were of interest but I knew most of it."* Two surgeons commented that they did not feel there were any courses targeted specifically to their needs.

4.2.8   Hospital meetings

Hospital meetings occurred at 15 of the 17 hospitals that the surgeons worked in. When surgeons did attend meetings they were appreciated as a learning tool. Although several surgeons commented on the advantage of having to prepare material for these meetings, the majority of surgeons liked hospital meetings for the opportunity to receive feedback on their progress. *"We have a weekly interdisciplinary meeting at our hospital that is usually well attended. It is a chance to show your cases and get decent feedback although there are some of the seniors whose reactions are a bit predictable. It is also an opportunity to see how the other young consultants are doing."*

4.2.9 Mentorship

Mentorship was identified in one form or another by eleven of the 17 surgeons interviewed. For six of these surgeons, it was their best teaching and learning experience. **Getting help from senior colleagues is clearly the most important way in which surgeons affect the transition from residency/fellowship into independent practice.** *"When I was appointed I was expected to be the trauma expert right from the start. That was why they had employed me. Fortunately, I was only a short distance from my old professor and he was always happy to help me out. To start with I would send him some patients but as time went by I did more and more difficult cases myself. I guess I would talk to him on the telephone every week. I don't know how I would have succeeded without him."*

4.3 Starting independent practice today: a surgeon's educational needs and implications for a teaching organization

The commonest educational need expressed by this group of surgeons is the ability to talk with seniors about their clinical problems. Interactivity and discussion is what is most important to them. The vast majority of these interactions occur within the institution in which the surgeon is working but such advice may not always be available within a single institution. Educational organizations can facilitate the creation of Internet-based communities of practice, which allow interaction between surgeons from different hospitals. Such communities need moderation and providing this is a rate-limiting factor.

Fellowships remain important for a small number of surgeons. Fellows greatly value the experience and the **fellowships sometimes trigger a lifetime relationship with the sponsoring organization and with the surgeon at the fellowship centre.** *"My fellowship was the most important part of my clinical training. My teaching institute was mainly focused on elective orthopedics and oncology. My trauma fellowship exposed me to a whole new way of thinking about trauma. X was a truly inspirational leader of the fellowship program and he introduced me to the importance of teaching. I still have contact with him and will continue to do so."*

Current formal educational courses do not seem to be targeted at this group of surgeons: a principles level course is too basic for them and an advanced course does not seem to be recognized as a useful educational resource. **Since surgeons at this stage in their career value one-on-one discussion as their preferred way of learning, it may be that formal educational events are not best suited to their needs and could not be easily modified to suit preferences.**

The surgeons who were interviewed did not seem to be short of information. The use of the Internet and its associated search engines means that surgeons can access information freely at anytime. Problems exist in the selection of relevant information. **Educational organizations can greatly assist surgeons by giving them access to information that has already**

been assessed as relevant to their needs. *"There is never a problem in getting online to look up information about a patient's problem. The trouble is that there is too much out there and it's hard to get exactly where you need to go. The Academy site is the best for me and I rely mostly on the review articles."*

Journals are more important to this group than surgeons-in-training but some surgeons have difficulty in accessing anything except the abstract for cost reasons. Educational organizations can help surgeons access full journal articles by purchasing group access on their behalf.

4.4   The beginning of practice as remembered by surgeons who began independent practice 5 to 10 years ago: needs and implications for a teaching organization

Origin of interviewees

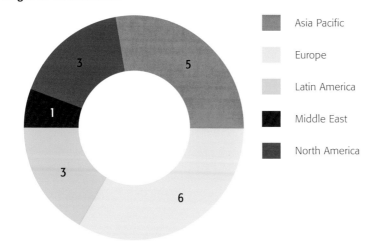

- Asia Pacific
- Europe
- Latin America
- Middle East
- North America

Eighteen surgeons who are currently acquiring expertise were interviewed for this part of the study. Five surgeons were from Asia Pacific, six from Europe, three from North America, three surgeons from Latin America and one surgeon was from the Middle East. The surgeons who were interviewed were between 5 and 10 years from the completion of residency. Two of the 18 surgeons interviewed continue to work under a degree of supervision at their places of residency. They had a degree of independent practice but still had to refer their decisions to the head of department.

The learning needs and preferences of surgeons who began their independent practice 5 to 10 years ago are broadly similar to those who are currently beginning this stage of their career. **Interactivity with friends and colleagues was historically a very important learning resource and still is.** There was a tendency for more people to be self-taught in this more senior group and there was a slightly heavier reliance on books. The Internet was the most important source of information for this group when they were after solutions to clinical problems but discussion with colleagues was the preferred learning route if this were possible.

The overwhelming majority of surgeons interviewed—13 of 18—felt that their typical learning experience had been interaction with people. Four of them described this as a clear one-on-one mentoring relationship and the rest had an informal network support usually within the institutions in which they worked.

One surgeon felt his typical learning experience was using books and another said his usual learning preference and typical learning experiences were using the Internet. Three surgeons felt that they were essentially self-taught at that stage in their career and all of those underwent a residency where they were given significant responsibility early in their residency. One surgeon commented, *"By the time I was appointed, I was used to doing things on my own so I didn't need much help from anybody."*

Ten of the surgeons interviewed felt that interaction with friends and colleagues was their best learning experience, four of whom described that relationship as being one of mentorship.

Four surgeons disagreed and felt their best learning experience was getting hands-on practice. *"Although I used to talk to colleagues for help, I never had a number one mentor. In the end, I learned by doing it."*

Three surgeons interviewed had become faculty members very early in their independent practice and all three of those rated their faculty membership as being their best learning experience. *"Being a faculty member meant that I had a network within the sponsoring organization which I phoned on a regular basis." "I was very lucky to be appointed to the faculty just before I was appointed as a consultant. My boss was the chairman of the course. Being a faculty member at such a young age was very important for me. It gave me status in my hospital when I was appointed. It gave me the chance to talk with very senior surgeons on an informal basis so I could discuss my problems."*

Interaction with people is the most important learning resource for this group of surgeons. The important relationships usually occurred within the institution that the surgeon worked in but others had more long distance contacts. Although none of the surgeons had a formal mentoring relationship with a colleague many of them had such a relationship even though it was not formalized. *"I now teach residents and we are assigned as a mentor to a resident. I even went on a course within my university to teach me how to do it. I never had that myself but looking back I see that my relationship with Y was very close to being mentored. It was all unofficial and down to Y's personality."*

Books formed a very significant learning resource for most of the surgeons interviewed. **Their use of books was more extensive than those who are currently at the beginning of their practice.** They relied on standard textbooks, and encountering clinical problems triggered use. This increased use of books does not appear to be linked to an inability to access the Internet.

One surgeon, who started in a fairly isolated practice in Latin America, said, *"Establishing a practice for me was very difficult. If it wasn't for the books, I don't know what I would have done. I then started to use courses as a way of learning how you should practice."*

The use of journals varied considerably within the group. Only five of the 18 surgeons identified journals a being a very important learning resource, whereas eleven felt that they were not very useful. *"Journals became very important to me as soon as I arrived in my new hospital. When I came across a new problem I often found I could not find the answer in a book. So I would go online and find out." "Journals were really not very useful. The research articles did not usually address my clinical problems. I found talking to my colleagues to be much more useful."*

When surgeons used journals, they accessed articles via the Internet. PubMed was the most common search engine used.

All but one of the surgeons interviewed used the Internet when they were beginning their practice. The one exception did not have access to the technology at that time. **All surgeons who used the Internet used it for communication, business, and for accessing information via search engines.**

The surgeons' interviewed were very divided in their opinions about how useful courses had been to them when they were starting their careers. Those who had not accessed courses during residency felt that these courses were useful.

The surgeons interviewed differed in their opinions about the importance of hospital meetings when compared to the surgeons currently starting their practice. **Nine of the 18 surgeons interviewed either did not attend hospital meetings on a regular basis or felt that they were very unimportant.** Six of the surgeons interviewed felt that regular hospital meetings were very important to them. Those who did value hospital meetings felt that it was the interactivity with colleagues which made it a successful learning experience.

Eight of the surgeons identified that they had a mentoring relationship while at the beginning of practice. Two of the surgeons interviewed had mentoring relationships as a result of a fellowship.

4.5   Beginning of practice as remembered by surgeons who began their independent practice more than ten years ago

Origin of interviewees

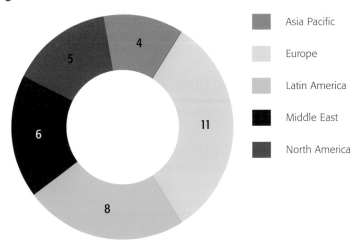

- Asia Pacific
- Europe
- Latin America
- Middle East
- North America

The surgeons interviewed varied considerably in their level of experience being between 10 and 30 years from the completion of their residency. Their memories therefore relate to sub specialty training between 1985 and 2000.

Thirty-five established experts in trauma surgery were interviewed. Eight surgeons were from Latin America, eleven surgeons were from Europe, and five surgeons were from North America. Six surgeons were from the Middle East and four surgeons were from Asia Pacific.

Established surgeons and surgeons beginning their independent practice had very similar responses about their best learning experiences during the post-residency stage of their careers. **Interactivity with friends and colleagues, especially if it is in the form of a mentoring relationship, was felt to be the most important aspect of their learning.**

Where their typical learning experiences differ is that many more experienced surgeons reported that their learning was primarily through on-the-job experience. As might be expected, books were more important to this senior group of surgeons. **The fact that none of these surgeons had access to the Internet is also a significant difference and as a result of this their use of journals varies considerably from the current cohort.**

Twenty-one of the 36 surgeons felt that their typical learning experience at the beginning of practice was learning by gaining experience on the job. These surgeons felt that they were self-taught and that they learned from their experiences in treating patients. This percentage of surgeons is much higher than that reported by surgeons who are currently at the beginning of practice or by surgeons who were in that stage 5 to 10 years ago. *"You were not expected to ask for help. You had been appointed as a surgeon and you were expected to get on with it. Learning from your own successes and failures was how you got better and more confident."*

Thirteen of the surgeons felt that interaction with people was the typical learning experience of that stage in their career and seven of them described the key relationship as being that of mentorship. Although this percentage of surgeons is less than currently seen, it is still a very significant element in the typical learning pattern of surgeons at this stage.

Two surgeons felt that their typical learning experience was reading books.

Twenty-one of the surgeons felt that interactivity was the best learning experience at that stage, a figure that closely mirrors today's cohort of surgeons. A remarkable ten of those surgeons identified a single colleague with whom they had a mentoring relationship.

Only five of the surgeons felt their best learning was learning by experience. *"Although I learned a lot from B, I'm essentially self-taught. The regular meetings we used to have had fell aside due to the rearrangement of hospitals." "I started off as an assistant consultant. You could call for help but they never came. I was largely self-taught and in the end learning from your own mistakes is the best form of learning."*

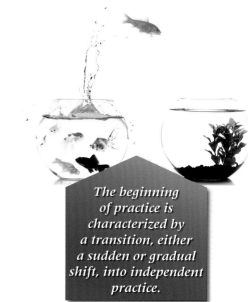

> The beginning of practice is characterized by a transition, either a sudden or gradual shift, into independent practice.

Three surgeons identified their best learning experience as attending a course. Two of these courses were in elective orthopedics. Two surgeons identified books as their best learning experience and three felt that attending congresses, both national and international, significantly helped their learning during the beginning of practice phase of their careers. *"Going to the state and national orthopedic meetings was the highlight of the year for me. You got to see your friends and talk to the experts. I always tried to do a talk or a poster which was another good way to force me to research, learn, and keep myself up to date."*

Interaction with people was the single commonest best learning experience of this group of surgeons when they were beginning their independent careers. Their pattern of response is very similar to the other groups of surgeons interviewed about their experiences. Informal mentoring was surprisingly common in this group of surgeons. Three of the mentoring relationships started as a result of fellowships.

Books were a very important learning resource for this group of surgeons when they were at beginning of their practice. Only two of the surgeons felt that books had not been helpful and **16 of the 36 surgeons interviewed felt that books had been incredibly important to them.** *"Right at the start of my career I would see a patient in the casualty department and examine him. I would then go back to my room and look it up in Campbell's. I would then go back to see the patient again, do anything that I had missed doing first time around, and then get on and treat him."*

As with other groups, the use of journals was very variable but most surgeons rated journals as being a very important learning tool. **This group of surgeons tended to use journals in a different way to the other groups examined because they did not have access to the Internet at this stage in their career;** none of the surgeons questioned had access to the Internet at the beginning of practice.

Journals therefore were accessed as printed material and not in an electronic format. Although the majority of surgeons still tended to look for journal articles in response to clinical problems, significant numbers of them subscribed to journals and read them on a regular basis. *"Every month the Trauma Journal would arrive and I would read it cover to cover. We did not have the Internet then and reading journals was the only way, apart from attending congresses, to keep up to date."*

Many of the surgeons interviewed did not have access to formal trauma courses during their residency and those that took courses during their beginning of practice rated them extremely highly. *"Well, I changed when I went on a course. Finally, I got to see how it might be done."*

There was a marked dichotomy of opinion with regard to how important meetings were as a learning resource when beginning independent practice. Nineteen surgeons rated hospital meetings as being very important. Those that valued the importance of hospital meetings felt it was due to the interactivity and the ability to get feedback from friends and colleagues. Eleven of the surgeons felt that hospital meetings were of no importance to them. The effect of this form of learning varied. *"Journal clubs were very confusing because I thought you could make the evidence fit any thesis."*

Eleven of the surgeons interviewed identified an informal mentoring relationship. As mentioned above, three of these were initiated as a result of fellowships. When mentorship was present, it was usually regarded by the surgeons as being their best learning experience.

4.6   How has the beginning of practice changed over time?

The beginning of practice is the most variable career stage studied. Two patterns emerge. The first is a dramatic shift from supervised residency to full independent practice. The second is a gradual change in the level of supervision leading over the years to full independent practice.

Both patterns of career have been present for a long period of time but there has been a gradual increase in the numbers of surgeons undergoing a more gradual transition into independent practice in the developed world. This change may reflect the increasing complexity of a surgeons practice and/or the decreased time available for training. Increasing numbers of surgeons are undergoing postresidency training and a more gradual transition into independent practice.

For both groups interaction, ideally on a one-to-one basis, with a senior colleague remains the most single important learning resource. The availability of these resources has become commoner with the passage of time. Formal mentoring is rare but informal mentoring is common and sought after. None of the surgeons had a mentor assigned to them at the start of their independent practice. The study cannot answer whether the development of such a system with adequately trained mentors would be welcomed by surgeons or whether this would result in improved patient care.

The increasing acceptance of seeking advice as the way forward for the young surgeon has been accompanied by a decrease in the number of surgeons who feel that learning by gaining experience on the job is their best learning resource. Gaining experience is a vital part of any surgeon's career but the pressure to just "get on and treat" appears now to be less than in the past.

The advent of the Internet has profoundly changed the way in which surgeons access information at the start of their careers. Journal articles remain as important as they have ever been but reading journals as opposed to accessing journal articles online is getting less common. The Internet rapidly became the most important tool for communication and information gathering almost immediately after its introduction. **Although access has become easier and faster problems with selecting relevant information remain.** The use of the Internet for eLearning does not appear to be relevant for surgeons when they are starting their independent careers.

Books have become less important as learning resources. Surgeons who began their independent practice 20 years ago relied heavily on books. The more modern generation is much less reliant. Books are now increasingly thought of as out of date.

Hospital meetings have become more important with the passage of time. They occur more frequently than in the past and are used not only for teaching but also for audit purposes. Supporting hospital meetings with relevant learning tools may be a desirable objective for a teaching organization.

Beginning surgical practice can be the most stressful stage of a surgeon's career. Existing educational resources do not seem relevant to the majority of surgeons interviewed. **Improved understanding of the educational requirements of this group of trauma surgeons could lead to the creation of more relevant educational resources,** such as communities of practice.

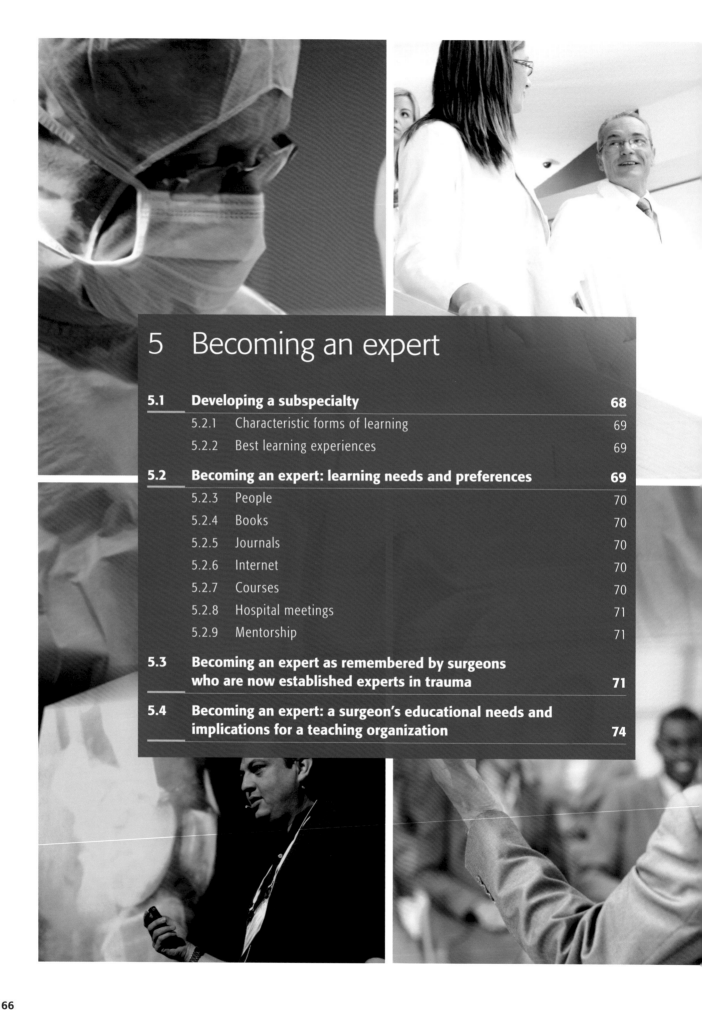

5 Becoming an expert

Chapter 5

Becoming an expert

As more senior surgeons describe learning experiences that have impacted them, a trend emerges; although the majority of learning may take place on-the-job, most identify interaction as the best way of gaining knowledge. This may indicate an opportunity for educational organizations to facilitate increased access to peers for case-based discussion.

Becoming an expert marks that period of time in a surgeon's career when he or she acquires expertise in a particular field of trauma or orthopedics. Surgeons interviewed have been in independent practice for 5-10 years. Two of the 18 surgeons interviewed continued to work under a degree of supervision at their places of residency. They had a degree of independent practice but still had to refer their decisions to the head of department.

Origin of interviewees

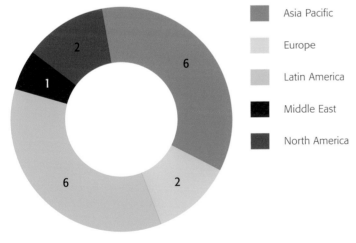

Asia Pacific

Europe

Latin America

Middle East

North America

Eighteen surgeons were interviewed who were between 5 and 10 years from the completion of residency. Five surgeons were from Asia Pacific, six from Europe, and three from North America. Three surgeons were from Latin America and one surgeon was from the Middle East.

5.1   Developing a subspecialty

Nearly all surgeons interviewed for this study chose to develop a specialist interest within the field of trauma and orthopedics. Forty percent of the surgeons interviewed decided to make trauma their specialist field. Sixty percent decided to specialize in a branch of orthopedic surgery. The commonest subspecialties were joint replacement surgery, hand surgery, and sports medicine. Many surgeons who specialized in trauma surgery commented that the majority of their colleagues had decided to specialize in a branch of orthopedic surgery and they felt in a minority. *"Most of my friends went off into other more lucrative branches of orthopedics like sports medicine. They think I am a bit mad to specialize in trauma but still seem quite willing to refer their problem cases on."*

The tendency to specialize in a branch of elective orthopedic surgery was much commoner in surgeons from the developed world. In the developing world trauma remains the dominant subspecialty within orthopedics and traumatology. *"Trauma is still the bread and butter of my practice. There is a never-ending supply of patients. Many of them have not been managed well by the doctor who saw them as an emergency, so there is plenty of secondary and reconstructive surgery to do. When the population becomes a lot older there will be a huge demand for joint replacement surgery."*

The start of this phase of a surgeon's career is variable. For surgeons in the developed world currently in training and those who completed residency within the last 15 years, the decision to subspecialize was usually made during the later stages of residency. Residents rotate through the subspecialties and get an opportunity to see what is available. Many also receive feedback as to their performance and suitability for specialty training. **For this group of surgeons who start their subspecialty training in residency, this phase of their career overlaps both residency and the start of practice phase. They do not experience a sudden transition** to a new phase in their careers and their education often begins in a formal way and may continue through a structured fellowship program. All current residency programs are trying to ensure that their trainees get exposure to subspecialties and the tendency to subspecialize earlier and earlier in a career is likely to continue.

The older generation of surgeons from the developed world and most current surgeons from the developing world start their subspecialization after the beginning of independent practice. Their transition into this phase of practice is more distinct but no surgeon interviewed described this stage of his or her career as being as stressful as the beginning of independent practice.

The choice of sub specialty is determined by many factors but patient demand and financial rewards are as important as aptitude in most surgeons thinking. *"There have been many advances in foot and ankle surgery in the last few years and patients who were treated non operatively are now starting to demand treatment. No one else in my hospital specialized in this type of surgery so I saw it as a great opportunity to establish myself in the community."*

The period of time taken to become an expert was variable with most surgeons taking 2 to 5 years. Most surgeons could not easily define an end point for this stage of their career. *"I wanted to become an expert in pelvic surgery and after taking a fellowship I joined an established practice to gain more experience. I guess it took about 3 years before I felt I had sufficient expertise to call myself an expert. That was the time I realized that other surgeons were referring cases to me by name as opposed to referring them to my unit. I don't think there will ever come a time when I don't have more to learn."*

5.2   Becoming an expert: learning needs and preferences

5.2.1   Characteristic forms of learning

The majority of surgeons (eleven of the 18) felt that their typical way of learning how to become an expert involved interaction with colleagues. Two surgeons identified a formal mentorship relationship but the majority felt that their relationship with colleagues was more informal and usually case based. *"When I decided that I wanted to specialize in joint replacement surgery I went on a company sponsored course to learn about how to insert resurfacing hip arthroplasties. When I was there I met a locally based surgeon who was part of the faculty. The company arranged for me to visit him to see him operate and subsequently he visited me. We often phone each other if we have unusual cases."*

Seven of the 18 surgeons said that learning typically occurrs merely by gaining experience in treating patients. *"I became interested in arthroscopy during my residency and made sure I did the right bit of the rotation to ensure I got the best training. I thought of doing a fellowship but did not have the time. I started doing simple procedures like removal of loose bodies and excision of bucket handle tears. Then as I got more experienced I started to do ACL replacements on a regular basis. I had learned the technique as a resident. Now I think I do a good job."*

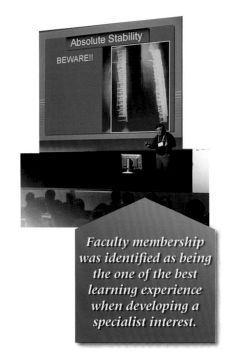

Faculty membership was identified as being the one of the best learning experience when developing a specialist interest.

5.2.2   Best learning experiences

Twelve of the 18 surgeons interviewed were already faculty members on educational courses and for this group, faculty membership was extremely important in meeting their learning needs. **Eight of them identified faculty membership as being their best learning experience when developing their specialist interests.** Two reasons were put forward for the success of faculty membership as a learning experience. Firstly, work is required to prepare to be a teacher at individual events, and secondly, interactivity occurs while on a course. *"It is the highlight of my professional year. I get to meet all my old friends and have a chance to talk through what has been happening. You get a chance to listen to experts talking about the latest developments. At the end of the day or during the coffee breaks there are always X-rays being handed around. You also have to do a presentation and of course you want to look good so you take some time to look things up and make sure you are up-to-date."*

Although most surgeons who are faculty commented that interactivity with peers and visiting experts was important, they also commented that the interaction between themselves and the course participants was a very important part in their own learning experience. *"I find I learn a lot from the participants. They often ask questions that I have never thought about and it is a great learning experience to have to answer them correctly."*

Only three surgeons who were faculty members did not rate their faculty experience as being very important to them. All three commented that they had joined the faculty as a career move and faculty membership was primarily useful to them in their career progression. *"I was pleased to accept the invitation to join the faculty but now attending the courses is not very enjoyable. I find it hard to justify being away from my very busy practice for such a long period of time."*

Of those members who were not faculty, all but one rated their best learning experience as interaction with colleagues. One surgeon felt that Internet use was by far his most important and best learning experience.

In summary, 17 out of 18 surgeons interviewed felt that interaction with peers (seniors or juniors) was their best learning experience during specialist training.

5.2.3 People
Interaction, whether through informal contacts within the hospital, or through educational organizations was the most highly rated educational resource by this group of surgeons. *"If I get in trouble, I phone some of my old colleagues in the UK." "Going to watch somebody and having the ability to discuss cases with him is the best part for me."*

5.2.4 Books
Textbooks seem significantly less important to this group of surgeons than to surgeons during residency or at the beginning of their practice. Ten of the 18 surgeons felt that books were of very little value to them and only five surgeons use books on a regular basis. *"Textbooks are no good if you are trying to keep yourself up-to-date. They are expensive and by the time they are published they are often out of date. Going to annual meetings is the best way of staying current."*

5.2.5 Journals
Journals were also not rated very highly by the majority of surgeons. All the surgeons accessed journals through the Internet and the majority accessed journal articles using a search engine, of which Google and PubMed were the most commonly used. Two of the surgeons regularly read journals online, but the rest accessed journal articles only if they had specific clinical problems.

5.2.6 Internet
All surgeons interviewed used the Internet. All surgeons felt that the Internet was their most important communication and business tool. Eight of the surgeons rated it as also being a very important learning tool for themselves. The reasons they accessed the Internet were consistent. Surgeons accessed information on the Internet if they came across a clinical problem or if they were preparing for an educational course, hospital meeting or national/international congress.

5.2.7   Courses

The majority of surgeons did not rate attending formal education courses as being important to their development as specialists. Surgeons who rated courses as being important referred to non-trauma related courses, for example arthroscopy and joint replacement courses.

5.2.8   Hospital meetings

Hospital meetings seemed to be less important to this group than to those undergoing residency or who were at the beginning of practice. There was, however, a dichotomy of responses—most surgeons felt such meetings were unimportant but a few surgeons rated regular hospital meetings as being important for feedback and quality control.

5.2.9   Mentorship

Mentorship in a formal sense is unusual in this group of surgeons. Only two surgeons identified a mentor and in both of those cases the mentoring relationship began with a fellowship.

5.3   Becoming an expert as remembered by surgeons who are now established experts in trauma

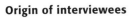

Origin of interviewees

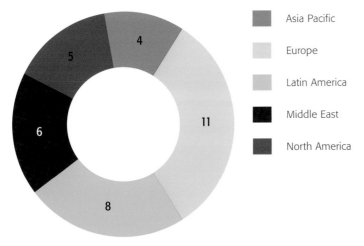

- Asia Pacific
- Europe
- Latin America
- Middle East
- North America

Thirty-five established experts in trauma surgery were interviewed concerning their experiences when they were acquiring knowledge to achieve specialist status. Eight surgeons were from Latin America, eleven Surgeons were from Europe, and five were from North America. Six surgeons were from the Middle East and four surgeons were from Asia Pacific.

The surgeons interviewed varied considerably in their level of experience. Interviewees were between 10 and 30 years from the completion of their residency. Their memories therefore relate to subspecialty training between 1985 and 2000.

Although many of the surgeons interviewed said that interest in their chosen subspecialty began while they were residents, **the majority felt that their training to be an expert occurred when they were in independent practice.** This is different from the younger group of surgeons whose subspecialty training began at a much earlier stage in their careers.

There were two main reasons for the differences. Firstly, residency programs 20 to 30 years ago were not as well structured as they are today. Secondly, the growth of subspecialization has increased rapidly over the past 25 years. The generalist orthopedic surgeon was the norm in the 1970s but is now virtually unknown in the developed world.

Many of the surgeons practiced at the time when subspecialization began and indeed some of them were pioneers in their fields. This may partially explain why many of them felt that they had essentially been self-taught. Educational resources were much less available. The Internet either did not exist or was in its infancy and the subspecialties themselves were just developing.

Although the start of specialist training differed from surgeons who are training to become experts today, the responses of the more senior surgeons were in some ways very similar to today's cohort when asked about their learning preferences. There were, however, some significant differences reflecting the advent of the Internet and development of the subspecialties themselves.

Thirty of the 35 surgeons described their typical learning experiences as acquiring knowledge through experience. Six of this group expressed the belief that they were entirely self-taught. *"I learnt from my own experience. Books are where you start from, then journals, and then the Internet." "We just started to use the Internet as a source of information but nothing beats just getting experience. I had two close colleagues who helped me but no mentors."*

Twelve of the expert surgeons said that becoming a faculty member on an educational course was their best learning experience; this is a consistent sentiment with surgeons who are currently training to become experts. Eighteen of the 36 surgeons were faculty members. It is clear therefore that surgeons who acquired faculty status during this stage of their career hugely valued this educational experience. When questioned, all faculty members felt that the interactions between faculty members and participants were why they regarded the faculty experience as being so rewarding. Two-thirds of the faculty members also added that they appreciated the stimulus to keep themselves up-to-date when given assignments as faculty.

Eight surgeons felt that discussions with colleagues were their best learning experience. This preference was very similar to that expressed by surgeons who are currently becoming experts.

Five of the surgeons felt that attending educational events was their best learning experience. The events were not educational courses: four of the five identified national or international congresses as being their best learning experiences.

Four surgeons felt that learning by doing was their best learning experience. All of these surgeons had been in independent practice for more than 25 years. **As with the younger group of surgeons there is a marked difference between the surgeon's description of typical learning—experience— and their description of best learning—interaction.**

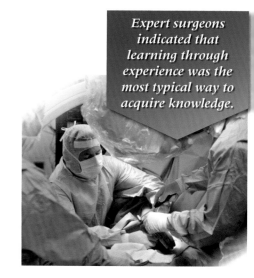

Expert surgeons indicated that learning through experience was the most typical way to acquire knowledge.

Interaction with other members of staff in their hospitals was an important learning resource for many of the surgeons questioned. The tendency to use colleagues as a learning resource was slightly less in those surgeons who are now experts compared to surgeons who are now acquiring expertise in their subspecialty. This could reflect a change in the willingness of surgeons in practice to ask for help and advice or merely reflect the decreased availability of expert advice when the subspecialties were developing.

Books were an important learning resource for this group. Older surgeons tended to use books more in their acquiring expertise career phase. In common with today's cohort, they valued journals more than books. The increased use of books may well be explained by the lack of the Internet when most of these surgeons were acquiring expertise.

Most of the surgeons did not have access to the Internet when they were becoming experts. They relied much more heavily on reading journals to keep up-to-date and to acquire expert knowledge. They tended to subscribe to journals and then read them on a selective basis. They did not have access to search engines and relied on library searches using indexes to find clinical problem solving information. Because of the difficulties in doing this many surgeons read journals "cover to cover". **A common use of journals was therefore keeping up-to-date rather than investigating specific clinical problems.**

The Internet was a very popular resource for those expert surgeons who had access to the Internet while they were acquiring expertise. It is not surprising that their use of the Internet was less than the current cohort, and as with all groups there were individuals who struggled to use the Internet. *"I don't use the Internet much except for communication. I find it's a lot faster to get information by reading a book."*

Attending formal educational courses was an educational resource that was used by comparative few of the surgeons questioned. **Surgeons could not identify courses that were useful to them when they were developing their expertise in trauma surgery.** Those surgeons who did mention attending successful courses usually referred to specialist courses outside the field of trauma.

Hospital meetings were a very important learning resource for this group of surgeons. The senior group of surgeons interviewed rated meetings as more important than the current cohort. Surgeons felt that hospital meetings were most successful because of their interactivity.

Mentorship was extremely unusual in the phase of developing surgical expertise trauma. Only two surgeons identified that they had a clear mentor figure through this phase of their career. In both cases, this relationship started as the result of a specialist fellowship.

5.4   Becoming an expert: a surgeon's educational needs and implications for a teaching organization

Interaction with peers and experts is both the commonest and pre-ferred way in which surgeons acquire expertise within the field of trauma. Surgeons who are currently developing specialist expertise and those who are established experts rate faculty membership as being their most important learning experience. They value motivation given by faculty membership in making them prepare presentations, etc. and they also hugely value the interactivity with peers, experts, and participants that take place during educational courses.

The majority of faculty members are extremely happy with their faculty experience but consideration could be given to **enhancing the faculty experience.** This could be done in a variety of ways. Interactivity with experts and peers could be facilitated by reserving a small part of the course time for a faculty-only event focused on a specific clinical problem. Such an event could be moderated by an acknowledged expert and consist largely of interactive discussion around prepared cases.

Setting up community of practice websites could also facilitate inter-activity. Any faculty member could post a case online, invite comments, and surgeons could interact about cases. Alternatively, regular virtual meetings focusing on one clinical area could be held by the group. Such meetings would be moderated by an expert and might include a didactic presentation as well.

Conventional books seem not to have a huge place in the learning framework of a developing specialist in trauma. Accessing information via a search engine on the web seems to be by far the most popular way of accessing material when a clinical problem is encountered. In general terms, surgeons prefer the Internet to books or journals when trying to solve unique clinical problems. Many surgeons comment that they find it difficult to access the information they require using the conventional search engines. **Teaching organizations could therefore consider setting up specialist sites whose contents were selected by appropriate experts.** Surgeons comment that they do not have a problem in accessing information but they do have a major prob-lem in selecting which information to access. Immediate access to a small number or relevant papers, videos etc. is preferable to accessing a long list of possible relevant sources.

Formal education courses do not seem to form an important part of a surgeon's development at this stage in his career. Faculty membership is very important, but surgeons at this stage do not report that there are successful courses designed with them as participants as opposed to faculty members. Surgeons who are becoming experts are very busy. They struggle to find time to access education and this is particularly true if they are a faculty member and need to take time off work to attend the course. Surgeons feel that their needs are usually focused around a particular clinical problem and that existing courses are too broad in their scope for them to benefit. **Short, expert only, highly interactive courses, focused on specific areas of clinical needs may represent a way forward.**

Although mentorship in a formal sense is rare at this stage of career development, it should be noted that four of the surgeons interviewed identify the fellowship experience as being the start of their specialization. Although only a small number of surgeons who take a fellowship sponsored by an educational organization will subsequently help that organization in its teaching activities, those who do so are very committed and dedicated contributors.

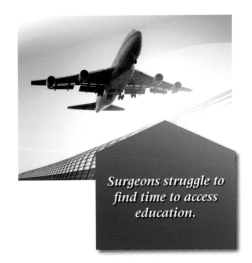

Surgeons struggle to find time to access education.

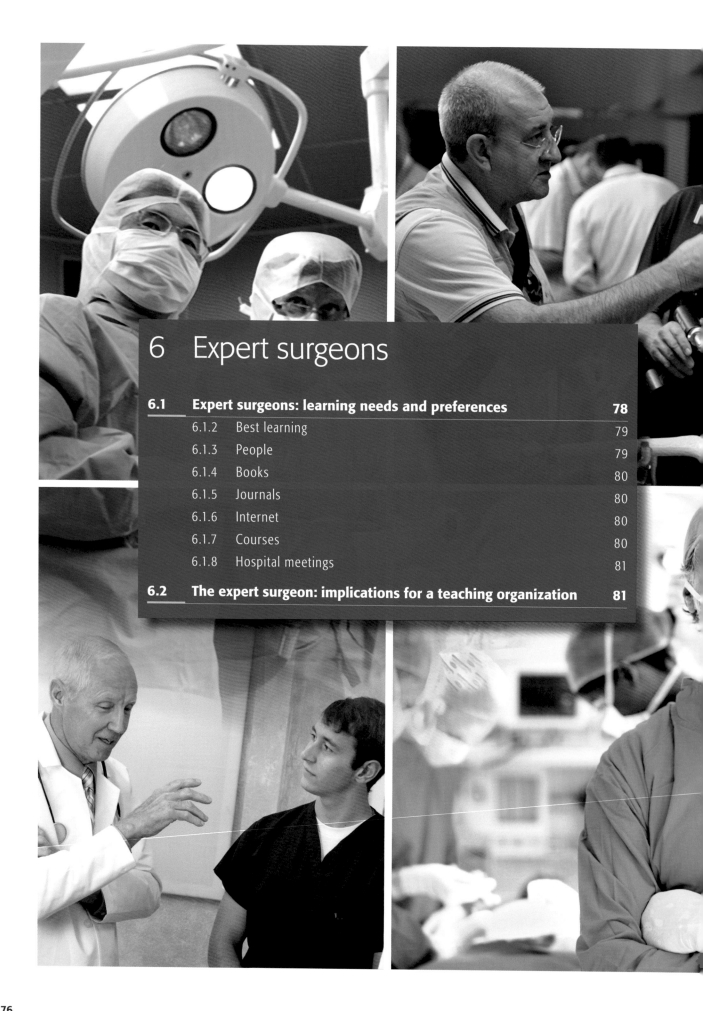

6 Expert surgeons

Chapter 6

Expert surgeons

Even after being in practice for over 10 years surgeons are reluctant to identify themselves as experts—there is always something new to learn. This group is more likely to be involved in research at the leading edge of science, gathering information from patient outcomes. A portion of this group identified being a faculty member on a trauma course as being their best learning experience.

Origin of interviewees

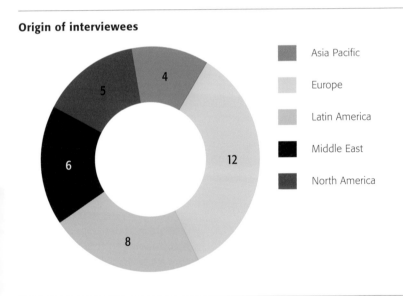

Asia Pacific

Europe

Latin America

Middle East

North America

Thirty-five experienced expert trauma surgeons were interviewed for this part of the study. All surgeons were at least 10 years from the end of their residency and had been in independent practice between 10 and 30 years. Twelve surgeons were from Europe, five were from North America, and eight were from Latin America. Four surgeons were from Asia-Pacific and six were from the Middle East.

All surgeons in this section of the study had developed a specialist interest within the field of trauma and orthopedics. Sixty percent of them had developed a specialist interest in trauma, which is a relatively high number when compared to the orthopedic specialty as a whole. This figure reflects the fact that the surgeons, although chosen at random, were picked from a list of surgeons who were known to have at least some interest in trauma. Surgeons with a low interest in trauma would have had no contact with the sponsoring body and would not have been available for interview.

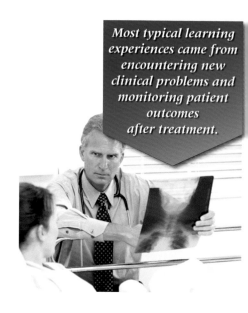

Most typical learning experiences came from encountering new clinical problems and monitoring patient outcomes after treatment.

Some of the surgeons described themselves as experts but many were reluctant to use that word. These surgeons felt that they still had a lot to learn and were continuing to develop as an expert. Very few felt that they had reached a plateau in their learning. *"I suppose my colleagues regard me as being an expert in lower limb reconstruction but I don't think of myself in that way. I seem to be continually discovering things and changing my practice. I don't think I will ever feel that there is not a lot more to learn."*

Whatever their learning styles or preferences the main reason that the experts looked for education was meeting a clinical problem. A typical response is embodied in the following from a surgeon from the Ukraine. *"Why do I look for education? Usually it is because I come across a problem I don't know how to solve. For years all we had were some old Russian textbooks and it was hard to change. Now we have access to the Internet and more chances to travel so I can find solutions to my problems."*

6.1   Expert surgeons: learning needs and preferences

6.1.1   Characteristic forms of learning
Of all the groups examined in this study, experts were most reliant on learning by experience. When asked to describe their typical learning experiences 21 of the 36 surgeons interviewed said that they gained knowledge as a result of treating patients. Most of their learning happened as a result of meeting new clinical problems and learning from how the patients did as a result of treatment. This form of learning was not associated with surgeons of a particular age or experience and was as common in the developed as the developing world.

Experts are often at the cutting edge of advances in surgery. Many are pioneering new methods and many are involved in trials to clinically evaluate new therapies. Sources of information that are relevant to their work may be difficult to identify and may indeed be absent. These factors may partially explain their typical learning behavior.

A senior academic surgeon from the developing world articulated another possible reason for this learning style. *"I am the professor and people look to me to provide answers. Within my own unit I sometimes feel isolated. In the end I always look to my own experiences when asked to provide help. Articles are good but there is nothing to replace your own experiences."*

Four surgeons described their typical learning experiences as teaching. All were in academic institutions and two of four surgeons were faculty members on trauma educational courses. *"Most of my learning now occurs when I attend our local trauma course as a faculty member. We usually have one or two outside experts who join the faculty and I learn a lot from their lectures and from being able to speak with them."* *"Every day in my unit we have a conference where every case done the previous day and every case that is scheduled for surgery today is discussed. I try to quiz the residents about why they are proposing a particular form of treatment and very often I find it gets me thinking about why we do things. Discussions with a group of keen, well-read residents is a good stimulus to keeping up-to-date and developing your own ideas."*

Three surgeons described their typical learning experiences as research. All three were working in academic institutions and all three referred to clinical rather than basic scientific research. One said their typical learning experience was attending hospital meetings, one surgeon said that his typical learning experience was reading books, and a third from a politically isolated country said that his typical learning experience was travelling to meet other surgeons. *"It is very hard to get visas to travel in and out of my country. Foreign visitors are often reluctant to come. So I try to travel once or twice a year to see another surgeon work in his clinic. Over the years I have built up a network of colleagues to visit, many of whom are immigrants from my country now living in the United States."*

In general terms, our experts stated that the majority of their learning takes place as self-directed learning based on the experiences that they gained in treating patients.

6.1.2   Best learning

Although the typical learning experience described by the senior surgeons was gaining experience by treating patients, their best learning experiences nearly all significantly involved interaction, of which the single most important type was membership of a faculty. **Fourteen of the 36 surgeons interviewed said their best learning experiences were being a member of a trauma course faculty.** Only five surgeons who were faculty members did not state that faculty membership was their best learning experience. *"I learned the skills of teaching and learned trauma as a result of teaching it."*

In common with all the other groups who included faculty members, they described two main reasons why faculty membership is so important to them. The first is that it gives them a stimulus to learn. The second is the interaction that takes place during the educational event. *"It is a great honor to join the faculty. I love the interaction as a faculty member. It is the personal contacts that have helped me most." "You surround yourself with people who have ideas of their own. I do most of my learning on courses at the back of the room talking to my friends when the lecture is going on."*

Three surgeons felt that attending national and international meetings was their best learning experience. Four surgeons stated that visiting friends or colleagues by travelling was their best learning experience. *"You can get a lot from books and even more from a discussion but the way you find out how things are is to visit someone in their clinic and watch what really happens. I went to Paris a number of years ago because I had heard that someone there was able to successfully treat patello-femoral arthritis. After watching him I realized that this would not work, at least in my hands. There is often a difference between a surgeons publications and the reality of his practice."*

Two surgeons felt that searching the Internet was their best learning experience. Two stated that reading journals was their best learning experience and one surgeon stated that doing clinical research was his best experience.

6.1.3   People

Learning by interacting with other people in the place of work was much less important to this group of surgeons than any other group. Only seven surgeons described this as being very important. It appears that interaction within their work environment is not important to many surgeons but interaction as a faculty member certainly is.

6.1.4 Books

Books were much less important than any other group studied; only nine surgeons regarded books as being very important. *"Books really don't give me what I'm after. They always seem to be out-of-date. The only books I still refer to are the classics such as the Letournel's Book on Acetabular Fractures."*

When surgeons use books they tend to rely on classic texts to remind them of particular points nearly always related to a clinical problem.

6.1.5 Journals

Reading journals is not important to this group of surgeons. Having said that, it must be remembered that reading journal articles by accessing them via Internet search engines is a very important source of information to them. Only five surgeons interviewed regularly subscribed to a journal and read it on a regular basis. All others only read journal articles if they were led there via a search engine.

6.1.6 Internet

The Internet was, in common with all groups, the most frequent way in which information is accessed. This was true for surgeons of all ages and from every country. All surgeons interviewed accessed the Internet on a regular basis and used it as their major communication and business tool.

Four surgeons tried to avoid using the Internet if possible. *"Finding stuff on the Internet takes far too long. If I got a problem and I can't answer, I know exactly where to find it in my library."*

Another major use of the Internet was to prepare themselves for teaching as faculty. Half of the faculty members mentioned that they used the faculty resource support packages on a faculty support website and found them to be very helpful.

6.1.7 Courses

Although experts experienced interaction with peers, colleagues, and seniors in several ways. They did not feel that there were any courses currently available which met their needs as learners. When asked why they do not regard existing courses as useful, several comments were made: *"If I attended a course, I want it to be focused purely on a single clinical issue that it is relevant to me." "I cannot afford 3 to 4 days off work at a time, particularly as I'm already giving that time to be a faculty member. If I were to be on a course, it would have to be 1 or 2 days at the most."*

Acquiring CME accreditation points did not seem to be important for expert surgeons. *"I did a one-day course that was not accredited. It was organized at a very nice hotel by a commercial company and taught me the skill that I was trying to acquire."*

This surgeon from the United States expressed the majority view. *"Yes, CME is important but I can pick up my points very easily. If I go to an educational event I go because I need to find out how to treat my patients and not because I need the points."*

6.1.8   Hospital meetings

There was a marked dichotomy in the responses with regard to how important hospital meetings were to learning when you were an expert. Many surgeons regarded hospital meetings as being irrelevant whereas others felt equally passionately that it was a very good way of interacting with people. Surgeons who worked in academic institutions felt that hospital meetings were of critical importance to ensure quality control within the units in which they worked.

No surgeon who is currently an expert identified a mentoring relationship as being in any way important to him or her at this stage of his or her career.

6.2   The expert surgeon: implications for a teaching organization

Thirty-one of the 35 surgeons interviewed described some form of interaction with other surgeons as being their best learning experiences. The commonest way of obtaining this interaction was as a faculty member. It must be remembered that the views expressed come from a highly selected group of surgeons. To be contacted in the first place, surgeons must have, at one stage, had a connection with the sponsoring organization. To respond, they must have had motivation to do so and therefore this group of responses represents a group of surgeons who are already largely committed to the sponsoring organization's model of teaching and education. Many of the interviewees were faculty members whereas most expert surgeons practicing in the world do not have any formal teaching commitments. What conclusions can be drawn from their strongly held view that teaching on an educational course is their best learning experience?

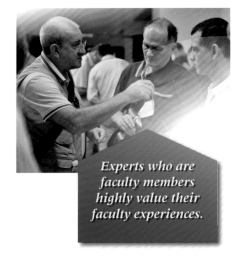

Experts who are faculty members highly value their faculty experiences.

This study has clearly shown that surgeons of all ages value interaction as part of their learning experience. Surgeons achieve this in a variety of ways dependant on their culture and seniority. Junior surgeons clearly cannot be faculty members because they lack the experience so this opportunity is only open to more senior surgeons. Junior surgeons frequently utilize a mentoring relationship to facilitate their learning but such opportunities, which usually take place with a more senior surgeon, are therefore usually not available to expert surgeons. Hospital meetings provide interaction between surgeons of differing experience but do not usually provide peer interaction for expert surgeons. These factors could explain why those experts who are faculty members value their faculty experiences so highly.

Could a learning organization facilitate peer interaction in another way? The advent of the Internet gives the possibility of long distance interactivity between expert surgeons. Such interactions would always be less effective than face-to-face discussions but would involve less time and would enable larger numbers of surgeons to get involved. Creating and facilitating such a network would appear ideally to be a task for an existing professional association with sufficient reputation to inspire confidence. This study has shown that a small number of surgeons feel that asking for help from a colleague is difficult.

Expert surgeons who are already faculty members consistently rate their faculty experience as being their best learning experience. They value the camaraderie, the interaction with experts, as well as their interaction with participants. Consideration may be given to enhance their faculty experience. Two surgeons started that while teaching a course they would like the opportunity to look at a particular subject in depth during a faculty-only session led by an acknowledged expert.

No educational organization currently provides education in the form of courses, which is felt to be suitable by expert surgeons. The surgeons commented that existing courses are too diffuse and last too long. It must, however, be remembered that the surgeons who were interviewed are nearly all trauma experts as opposed to orthopedic experts who do trauma.

Experts use the Internet as their major source of information and employ standard search engines. Surgeons do not have difficulty in accessing information but do have problems in information overload and the lack of selectivity of the existing search engines.

Teaching is an important part of the job for many surgeons interviewed. Five of the interviewees had taken faculty development courses and all were very positive about their experience. The faculty development program is primarily aimed at improving teaching on courses. **However, the skills acquired during faculty development are of considerable value to those surgeons who are involved in teaching on a day-to-day basis in their place of work.**

The surgeons interviewed did not readily identify books as being a useful source of learning to them as experts. When they did use books it was to gain reference from classical textbooks. **The non-library market for specialized textbooks therefore seems to be limited.**

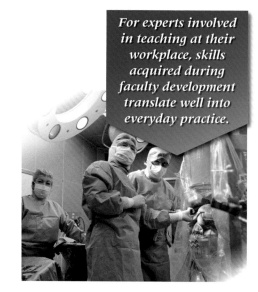

For experts involved in teaching at their workplace, skills acquired during faculty development translate well into everyday practice.

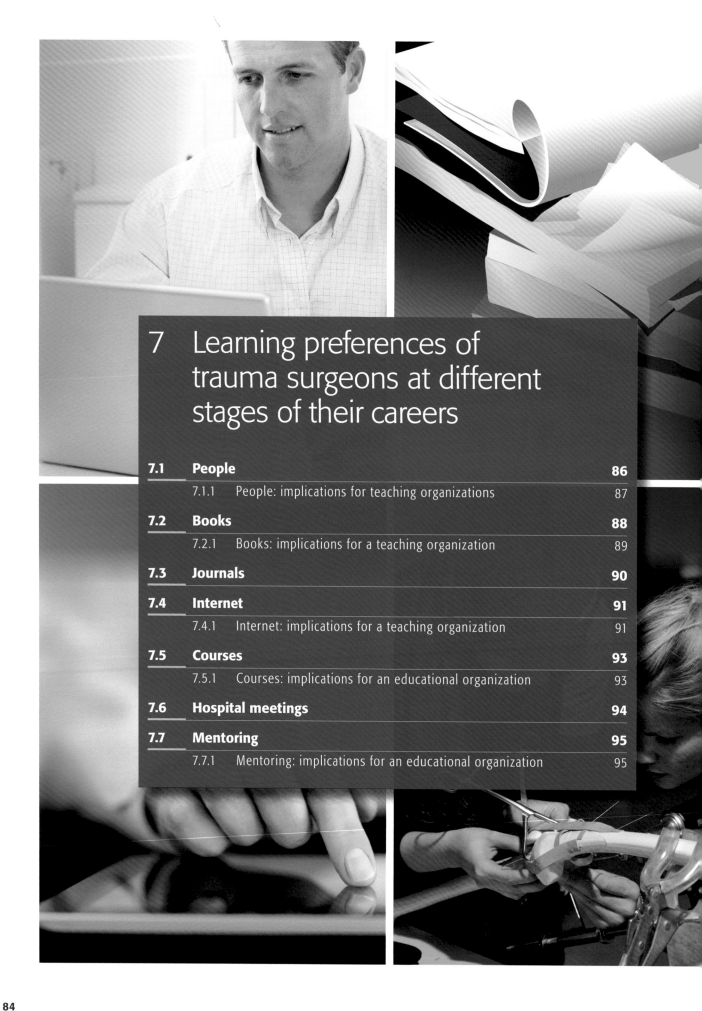

7 Learning preferences of trauma surgeons at different stages of their careers

Chapter 7

Learning preferences of trauma surgeons at different stages of their careers

Visual representations of the data gathered in the study display a pattern of learning that evolves throughout a surgeon's career. Learning resources that are important to a resident are not necessarily valued in the same way by an expert surgeon, and vice versa. A significant area for development lies in the realm of the Internet and its ability to connect people across distances when most convenient for them.

This study interviewed surgeons at all stages in their careers and asked them their current educational preferences and past experiences. The study was designed to provide an understanding about how educational preferences change over time as well as how educational preferences differ at each stage of a surgeon's career. This chapter will explore both aspects.

Graphs are shown to illustrate trends. They have been created from the data with a numerical score taken from the responses given by the surgeons. A best learning experience has been arbitrarily given a score of 5. Because the surgeons were not asked to score their preferences on a Lickert scale and the study was qualitative in design these numbers are not definitive. The pattern of responses shown in the graphs does, however, graphically illustrate many of the observations made by the surgeons.

7.1 People

Interaction with people is important to successful learning at all stages of a surgeon's career. However, the pattern of interaction varies considerably depending on the seniority of the surgeon.

Residents rate interaction with other members of the hospital team to be very important. Discussions with attendings or consultants are the most important interaction for residents but interactions with other residents, both peers and seniors, are also very important.

Historically, senior surgeons were often not present during parts of residency training and therefore interaction with senior residents, senior nurses, etc. was more important. There is evidence in this study that senior surgeons are now much more closely involved in residency training and have become an important learning resource.

Although many training schemes foster an active mentoring relationship between the trainer and trainee, very few of the interviewed residents identified a formal mentoring process as being any part of their current training.

Surgeons who are at the beginning of their independent practice report that interaction with people is by far their best learning experience. These relationships are significantly different from those described by residents. Surgeons at the start of independent practice tend to acquire a close one-on-one connection with a senior surgeon. This relationship often is de facto a mentoring relationship but nearly all these contacts are informal rather than formal. Many of these relationships start with a fellowship experience. The development and use of a mentoring relationship is a characteristic of learning in this group of surgeons and is almost unique to it.

Surgeons who are becoming experts rely less on interaction with people in their own hospitals. However, those who are trauma course faculty members hugely value interaction with fellow faculty members, experts, and participants, when present on a course. Mentoring relationships that formed in the beginning of the practice phase may continue when a surgeon is developing expertise, but mentoring as such becomes much less relevant during this stage of a surgeon's career.

Of all the groups examined, experts least rely on interaction with other staff members at the hospital. However, surgeons who are becoming experts and those who are faculty members hugely value the opportunity for interaction that comes as a result of being a faculty member. Senior surgeons often use interaction at hospital meetings as a form of quality control enabling them to understand what is going on in all parts of their units.

Importance of interaction with people at various stages of a surgeon's career

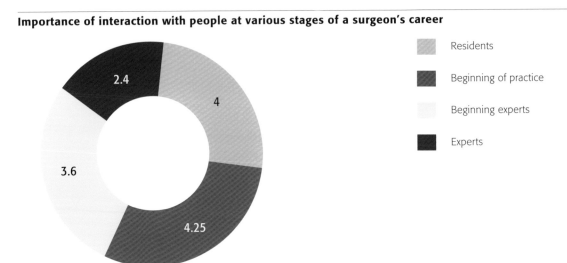

7.1.1   People: implications for teaching organizations

Teaching organizations increasingly focus on interaction within their courses rather than didactic presentations. To support this trend faculty members receive training in facilitating interactive discussion activities and these acquired skills can also be applied in the work place when interacting with other staff members. **Skills learned in faculty education programs that are applied in daily clinical practice** will facilitate meaningful interactivity with other staff members, making these encounters more productive for all.

Fellowships are sometimes the start of a long-term mentoring relationship between the trainer and the fellow. These relationships are infrequent but when they occur they can be very productive for the fellows and the patients they treat. **Trying to foster a continuing relationship through a network between the fellow and his fellowship hospital** is a possible way to make fellowship a more long-lasting and supportive experience.

7.2   Books

Books are important learning aids to trauma surgeons at all stages in their careers but distinct patterns of use emerge from this study.

Books are most important at the resident stage of a surgical career. Characteristically, residents buy standard textbooks at a very early stage in their residency and refer to them frequently at the start of training. The current cohort of residents-in-training report that they use books less as they progress through residency. They also report that whereas initially they read the book on a chapter-to-chapter basis as they became more senior they start to use books much more selectively usually on the basis of clinical problems that they had encountered.

The popularity of books as learning tools for residents has not really changed much in the past 20 to 25 years. The importance which current residents attach to books is almost identical to that reported by more senior surgeons when asked how important books were to them when they were in residency. **Despite the huge popularity and importance of the Internet, books remain an integral part of residency and there is no evidence in this study that as yet their popularity has significantly declined.**

As surgeons become more senior books become progressively less important to them. This pattern is again seen regardless of which cohort is examined.

Surgeons who are beginning practice use books significantly less than residents. They tend to use books relating to clinical problems and are less likely to browse.

Surgeons who are becoming experts or who already are experts use books even less. They comment that books are frequently out-of-date. If they do access specialist books, it is usually via a library. There seems to be a desire of senior surgeons to access the information that is in specialist books but this is not matched by a desire to purchase the books themselves.

At all stages of a surgeon's career surgeons refer (to a greater or lesser extent) to a relatively small number of classic textbooks, of which Campbell's, Rockwood and Green, and Hoppenfeld are the most frequently quoted.

Importance of books to surgeons at various stages in their careers

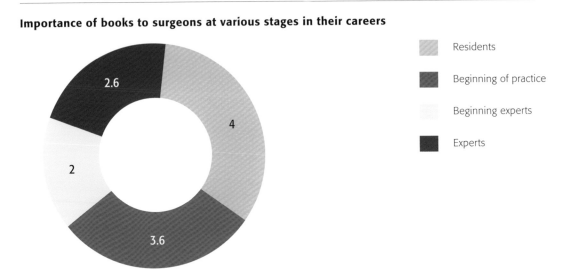

7.2.1   **Books: implications for a teaching organization**

Books are mainly used and valued by residents at an early stage of their careers. They still prefer a generalized text but as they become more experienced they use books in a different way—focusing on small sections of individual chapters that are relevant to the clinical issues they are facing.

Experts seem to want access to expert textbooks but when they do so, it's on a case basis. At present, there is a tendency for surgeons to use the Internet and access the information through articles. **If sections of specialist books could be available via an online search engine** then it is possible that many surgeons would access this information. Many of them commented that the journal articles which they are led to via Internet search engines may not be directly relevant to their patient's needs.

There is no evidence in this study that the need to produce textbooks whether in print or electronic format for the use of residents-in-training is in anyway declining with time. The way surgeons access books (print/electronic) will change radically but the need for standard textbooks appears to still be present. The role of textbooks as references and exam curricula guides should also not be underestimated.

7.3   Journals

Journal articles are the major source of new information for surgeons of all stages in their careers, except for junior residents who rely almost exclusively on textbooks. Although journal articles are always critically important for surgeons of all levels, reading journals becomes progressively less important as a surgeon becomes more experienced.

The use of the Internet has revolutionized the way in which journal articles are accessed and used. Historically, surgeons subscribed to journals or got their libraries to do so. They then selectively read articles from those journals triggered by their interests and the needs of their patients. However, for the last 10 years or so, access to journal articles has been via the Internet and usually takes place with one of the following three search engines: PubMed, Ovid, or Google.

Importance of journals to surgeons a various stages in their careers

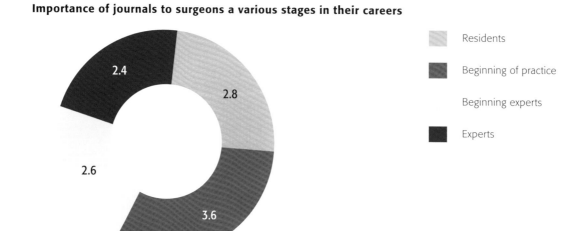

Residents

Beginning of practice

Beginning experts

Experts

7.4   Internet

The Internet is important to all groups of surgeons who were interviewed. There is a tendency for residents to use the Internet more frequently and more extensively than other groups but even the most senior surgeons rely heavily on it.

All groups use the Internet for communication and business as well as for gathering information. All groups tend to access information via a search engine and the commonest source of information is journal articles.

Curiously, although all surgeons use the Internet, enthusiasm for the Internet is surprisingly uncommon. The surgeons accept the Internet as a critical part of information gathering but few seem to relish its use.

Importance of the Internet to surgeons at various stages in their careers

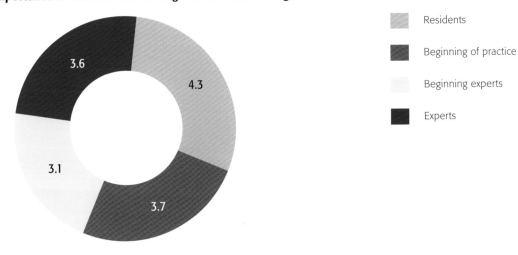

Residents

Beginning of practice

Beginning experts

Experts

7.4.1   Internet: implications for a teaching organization

There are several new uses of the Internet, which may be of significance in developing future educational strategies.

Three surgeons interviewed are members of an Internet based learning community. National orthopedic associations had set up two and the third occurred spontaneously within that surgeon's community. All three were extremely enthusiastic about this development and used their community membership to discuss clinical problems. All groups had discussions that were monitored and mediated by a senior surgeon. An orthopedic branch of Facebook has been set up by the Royal College of Surgeons in Edinburgh but no data about its use was available from the surgeons participating in this study. **The development of communities of practice,** which is relatively common in certain fields of medicine such as diabetes and nephrology, is a potentially exciting development for trauma surgeons and facilitating such groups **could be a future role for an educational organization.**

Surgeons vary considerably in their opinions about the existing search engines. Many find them satisfactory but there are common complaints that the information that they are led to is not necessarily the information that they need. **There is a general desire to access a smaller amount of relevant information rather than a huge amount of irrelevant information.** A possibility therefore exists to develop an information service which is selective and which will meet the surgeon's needs. There is no point in trying to develop a fully comprehensive search engine because these already exist. There may however be a need to provide surgeons with a filtered search engine, which will lead them to clinically relevant information.

The app is a relatively new development in web-based technology. Large numbers of residents particularly in the United States now use apps for a variety of tasks outside the field of orthopedics. Some US residents greatly value the idea of developing specialist apps targeted at specific clinical problems and to give them instant access to the information they need. Speed of access and accuracy are the two things that would be most valued in such a service. **Ensuring that all educational products are available on mobile devices is clearly essential for this group of surgeons.**

Although eLearning technology has been around for over 15 years, there is a surprising lack of use of this type of material by surgeons who took part in the study. Only two of them stated they regularly took part in self-directed eLearning activities and both of these were related to their training programs. The majority of surgeons seemed unaware of existing eLearning programs. More work needs to be done to find out why eLearning has not taken off in the way it might have been expected to. Understanding what makes the difference between successful eLearning and unsuccessful eLearning is critical for the development of new educational material.

Several of the surgeons interviewed stated that they valued video as an important and unique part of Internet-based learning. Curiously, YouTube remains their preferred source of videos.

Wheeless is an electronic Internet-based textbook that is frequently used by residents. It is valued because of instant access. The textbook itself only gives a small amount of bullet-point information about each topic and this is greatly valued by residents-in-training when preparing for trauma rounds, hospital meetings, etc.

7.5   Courses

Courses of all types become progressively less valued by surgeons as they become more experienced.

Courses are very important to residents-in-training and nearly all surgeons who have taken a principles level course report that it was a very good learning experience. Surgeons feel that a principles level course should be taken early in training. The practicals are the most valued part of the course. By the time surgeons enter more senior positions existing courses become less and less relevant. Experts complain that there are no courses specifically designed to meet the unique clinical problems they face, and there are also problems with regard to how long these events take.

Popularity of courses at various stages of a surgeon's career

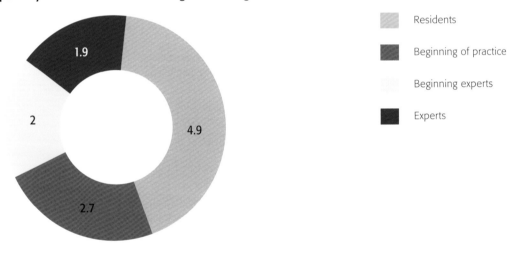

Residents

Beginning of practice

Beginning experts

Experts

7.5.1   Courses: implications for an educational organization
Residents value existing courses but they become much less popular and useful as a surgeon becomes more experienced.

If courses are to remain part of surgical education for senior surgeons they will need a radically different structure (see Chapter 6).

7.6   Hospital meetings

Hospital meetings vary considerably in their importance depending on the stage of career that the surgeon has reached.

Hospital meetings are very highly valued by residents–in-training. They like the interaction, the opportunity for discussion, and the chance to hear other people's opinion. They value the stimulus given to them by hospital meetings to prepare material. Although most surgeons at the beginning of practice value the opportunity to talk with seniors, hospital meetings do not necessarily give them that opportunity. Hospital meetings are more important for experts. At that stage, the majority of surgeons value hospital meetings as a good opportunity to understand what is going on in their unit and exercise quality control.

Importance of hospital meetings to surgeons a various stages of their careers

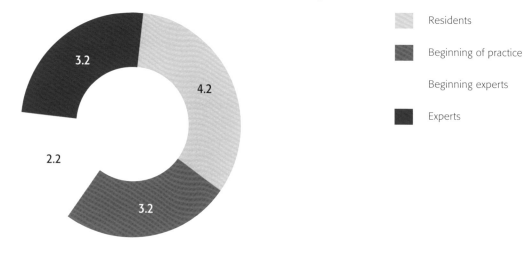

Residents

Beginning of practice

Beginning experts

Experts

7.7   Mentoring

Although formal mentoring was introduced into residency training a number of years ago, the only group of surgeons who report mentoring as an important part of their learning experience are those surgeons who are beginning their practice.

Entering independent practice for the first time is a very stressful experience for many people and the ability to discuss their problems with a more senior surgeon is highly valued.

Importance of mentoring to surgeons at various stages of their careers

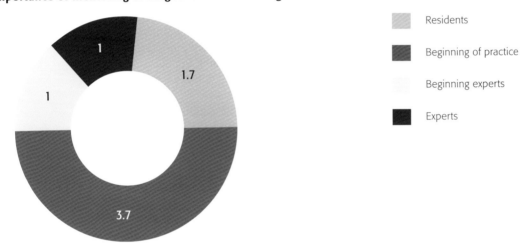

Residents

Beginning of practice

Beginning experts

Experts

7.7.1   Mentoring: implications for an educational organization

Mentoring relationships feature significantly at only one stage of a surgeon's career—the beginning of practice. Most of these mentoring relationships occur within a single institution and remarkably nearly all of them are informal. Some of the relationships identified in this study arose as a result of a fellowship. When this occurs, the relationship often continues for many years and as a result the surgeon often becomes very involved with the organization.

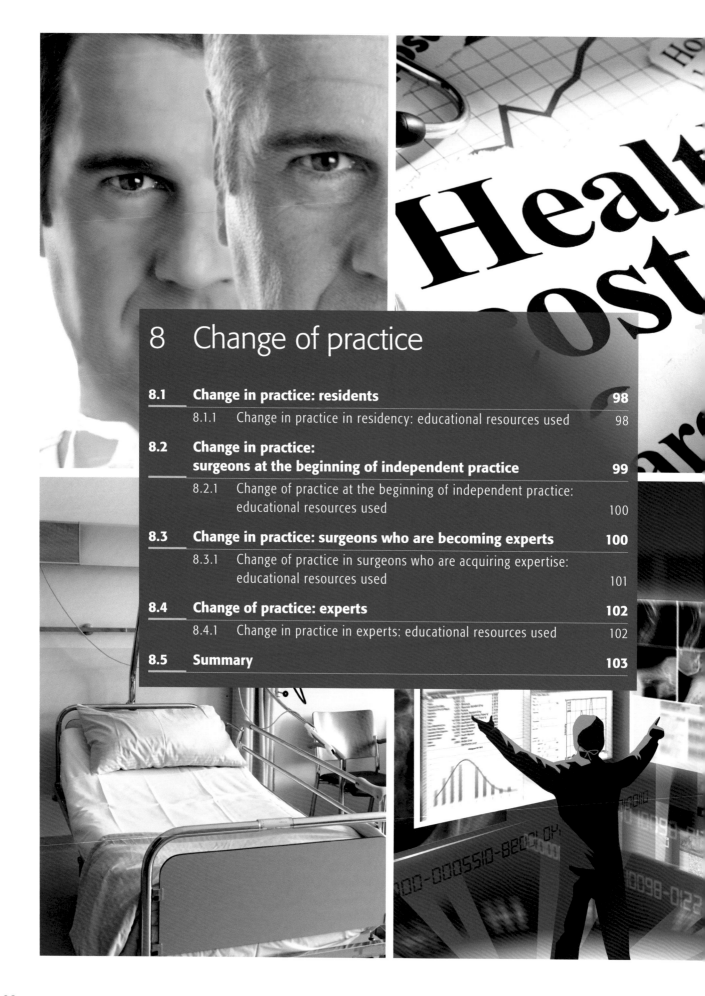

8 Change of practice

Chapter 8
Change of practice

The vast majority of interviewees had adopted a change of practice in the past year, regardless of their career stage. Motivation to do something differently was generally caused by concern for patient outcomes and the availability of new technologies. Education resources to support their changes were sourced from a variety of places but information supplied by commercial companies was the predominant reference.

At the end of each interview all surgeons were asked whether they had changed their practice in the last year. If they had, they were then asked why they had changed and what educational resources they had used to facilitate the change. Eighty-seven surgeons had made a change in the last year, 13 had not.

The most important reasons for a change in practice are remarkably consistent at every stage of a surgeon's career. Even in residency, where learning is driven by curriculum, it is evident that surgeons are driven to change practice for two main reasons:

- Change occurred because they encountered a clinical problem that was difficult to solve and required the acquisition of new knowledge, attitudes, and skills.
- Change was triggered by the development of an innovation: a new technique, procedure, or "trick" that they thought would help improve the outlook for patients.

The data presented in this section is directed towards investigating how surgeons learn and change the way they practice. The data was obtained both through the formal interview process and by surgeons volunteering information without prompting by the interviewers. The data is striking because although the reasons for implementing change are consistent throughout all stages of a surgeon's career, the ways in which change occurs vary considerably as the surgeons pass through different stages in their careers.

8.1   Change in practice: residents

Twenty-seven of the 30 surgeons said that they had changed some aspect of their surgical practice within the last 12 months. Of the three who had not changed their practice, one worked in a rural hospital in Africa and was unable to initiate the changes he wanted to because he did not have the resources. The other two said that they had not changed their practice because they had not become aware of any evidence that persuaded them to do so.

Of the 27 surgeons who had changed their practice in the last year, 16 said they had changed their treatment of patients because they had changed hospitals and/or consultants as a result of a rotation in their training program. *"When you change from one hospital to another, which we do every year, you have to get to learn how to use the implants available. Every hospital seems to have a different contract with a different supplier. It is very good for training because you get to make your own mind up as to which implants or techniques you are going to use when you become an attending."*

Even though these doctors do not have independent practice, six residents said that they had changed their surgical practice for clinical reasons. All six had become aware that certain aspects of their own clinical practice were, in their own opinions, not adequate and this was the reason they changed.

Four surgeons stated that their reason for change was that they had become aware of new technology. Three of these four referred to new implant technologies and the fourth to a new radiographic technique. The remaining surgeon who changed said that he did so as a result of his own experience and that he was developing his techniques to make his surgical approaches smaller and less destructive to the soft tissues. *"I read the literature on minimally invasive trauma surgery and realized I had been doing many things wrong. So I started to change."*

8.1.1   Change in practice in residency: educational resources used

When surgeons changed their practice as a result of changing their surgical rotations, nine of the surgeons said that the most useful educational resource enabling them to make the change was interaction with the senior surgeons who had introduced them to the new technology. One surgeon who had changed his practice as a result of changing rotations said that senior residents had been his major educational help. Five of these surgeons said that technique guides made available online by companies were their major educational resource and a single surgeon said that workshops organized by the implant manufacturer were of most use to him. The remaining resident who changed as the result of a rotation said that literature, mainly company literature, was his major educational resource. *"When the next group of residents starts in the hospital the industry representative organizes a workshop so we all know how to use the tools."*

When the group was studied as a whole, twelfe surgeons said that senior surgeons were the major educational resource helping them to affect change. Ten of the surgeons said that their major educational resources came from a commercial company. This help came from online technique guides, commercial company workshops, and consultants. One surgeon said that he was self-taught. One surgeon identified videos being his major educational resource and a final one said that exploring the Internet was his best educational resource. *"After I did a principles Course I rotated to pediatrics so I did not get to see an ankle fracture for 6 months. I used the video I had seen on the course to refresh my memory."*

It can be seen that changing rotation is a major driver for changing surgical technique in residents–in-training. This is of course not surprising. What is surprising is the vital role that company literature, technique guides, workshops, and sales consultants play in helping surgeons make these changes during their training. Although the majority of residents reported that it was interaction with their trainers that was their major resource, a large number of surgeons identified and **preferred information given by commercial companies that was targeted specifically at the techniques and skills required to change to new implants.**

8.2   Change in practice: surgeons at the beginning of independent practice

All 17 surgeons had changed some aspect of their surgical practice within the last year. Eleven of the surgeons changed their clinical practice in response to a clinical issue—usually a failure of treatment. Although the stimulus for change was usually a clinical issue, the majority of the surgeons were aware at the time they decided to change that there was new technology available, which gave them the possibility of improving patient care.

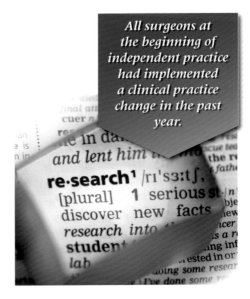

All surgeons at the beginning of independent practice had implemented a clinical practice change in the past year.

Three surgeons felt that advances in technology rather than an attempt to address a clinical issue drove the change that they had made. One surgeon went even further and said that his change in surgical practice was urged by peer pressure from his colleagues, who had adopted new technology with regard to the fixation of proximal femoral fractures. *"All my colleagues decided that they would treat all extra-capsular hip fractures with proximal femoral nails. I felt the evidence was not there to justify this change but did not want to be the odd one out."*

One surgeon said that his own study of the evidence led him to make a change with regard to the technique used for a particular fracture fixation. A final surgeon commented that he changed his clinical practice as a result of research.

8.2.1   Change of practice at the beginning of independent practice: educational resources used

Seven of 17 surgeons interviewed felt that implant manufacturers were the best learning resource when it came to affecting change. Of these, four surgeons said that their best learning asset with regard to achieving change was the help of a company representative and the other three surgeons felt that their best learning tool was information given out by implant manufacturers, accessed via the Internet. *"A company representative came around to see me with some new implants. I thought that they looked interesting and he then arranged for a workshop to be carried out in my hospital. After the workshop, I used the company's technique guides, which were online, to help me understand how to put these new implants into patients."*

Four of the surgeons felt that the change in their surgical practice had come about because they were self-taught. *"I'd heard a lot about minimally invasive techniques from my colleagues. It gave me the idea to start reducing the size of my incisions and I found that over the last year, I've been able to do a lot more through a lot smaller approaches."*

Two surgeons identified colleagues as being their major learning resource. Three surgeons identified the Internet as being their major source of educational health.

It seems that at the start of a surgeon's independent practice, his or her desire to change is usually triggered by clinical issues. The role of developing new technology is, however, huge and **the presence of new technology seems to bring to light perceived deficiencies in clinical practice.** The educational input of implant manufacturers is highly valued by most surgeons who participated in this study and the role of company representatives, technique guides, and other company literature should not be discounted when assessing the learning resources available to surgeons.

8.3   Change in practice: surgeons who are becoming experts

Experience of interviewees

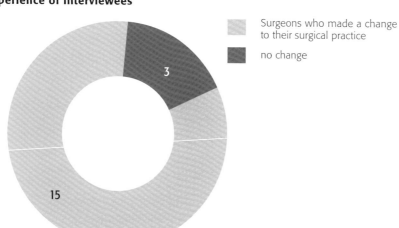

Surgeons who made a change to their surgical practice

no change

Fifteen of the 18 surgeons interviewed said that they had made a change in their surgical practice in the last 12 months.

Seven surgeons reported that the reasons for their changing practice were clinical issues that had arisen as a result of their existing practice. All of these surgeons had made a change in the way that they treat pathologies that have a poor prognosis. All of the surgeons reported that although the reason for changing their practice was based on clinical needs, they were aware at the time they initiated the change that newer techniques and technologies were available which might help their patients.

Four of the surgeons interviewed commented that their reason for changing was the advent of new technology. They had become aware of new technology through a variety of sources including advertisements, the literature, and visits from company representatives.

One surgeon went further with the following comment: *"I was visited by a company where they've showed me a new plate designed for the symphysis pubis. I had had problems with previous plates and so I used it. My experience was a disaster and four of the eight plates that I put in broke."*

Two of the surgeons interviewed said that their reason for changing practice was experience that they had gained on a short-term fellowship. One surgeon said that his change came about as a result of attending an educational course as a faculty member. A final surgeon commented that his reason for change was patient expectation. *"There was an article in our local paper about minimally invasive surgery in people who had had accidents. After that, patients came to see me and specifically asked if I was able to do these techniques. I got hold of some technique guides through various companies and was able to meet their expectations."*

8.3.1 Change of practice in surgeons who are acquiring expertise: educational resources used

Surgeons used a variety of educational resources to help them affect change.

Five surgeons used the resources provided by commercial companies— online technique guides, workshops and visits from company representatives. Three surgeons relied on scientific journals, which again they accessed online. Two surgeons identified being members of a trauma faculty as their best learning resource. One surgeon felt a website was his major educational resource. One surgeon identified visiting other clinics as being the most useful learning tool and two surgeons reported that conversations with their colleagues were the most important asset in letting them affect the change.

8.4   Change of practice: experts

Twenty-nine of the 35 surgeons interviewed said that they had made a change in their surgical practice in the past year. Seventeen of the 29 surgeons who had changed their practice changed for clinical reasons. **The commonest indication for change was the belief that the existing practice was inadequate to deal with certain types of pathologies.** The two commonest changes noted were the increased use of locking plates and minimally invasive techniques. Although surgeons who changed technique by changing implants did so primarily for clinical reasons, clearly all of them were aware that new technology existed which made the change possible.

Six of the surgeons interviewed felt that their stimulus to change was access to new technology. Surgeons became aware of new technology from a variety of sources, but the vast majority of them became aware through the action of the implant manufacturers. Advertisements in professional journals, visits from local sales representatives, and advertising delivered by mail were the major sources of this information. Two surgeons said that they became aware of new technology by reading scientific articles in journals and that that was their reason for changing their techniques.

Three consultants who were interviewed had to change hospitals and that led to a change in techniques. The response to a change in hospital was variable. One surgeon stated, *"The new hospital gave me daily trauma lists, which meant that I didn't have to get up at night to do surgery. It has completely changed my indications with regard to the timing of surgery for open fractures." "Moving hospitals was a very traumatic experience. I found that my new unit had a very high sepsis rate. I had to set about instituting daily trauma rounds and weekly morbidity and mortality conferences to ascertain the nature of the problem. A change in antibiotic prophylaxis in elective surgery resulted from these meetings."*

8.4.1   Change in practice in experts: education resources used
Surgeons gained information from a variety of sources. **The largest providers of useful information were the implant manufacturers.** Four of the surgeons said that technique guides, which were available to them online, were a major, helpful learning resource. Three surgeons attended company workshops. They recognized that these were not CME accredited events but felt that they were very helpful to them. In essence, they had already decided to make a change and the purpose of the workshop was merely to ensure they had the requisite skills required to make that change. Two surgeons felt that the local implant manufacture representatives were their major learning resource in making the change.

Three surgeons said their colleagues in their local hospital were their major learning resource. These could be either senior or more junior colleagues. One surgeon said, *"When the new surgeon came into town, he brought with him the new Expert Tibial Nail. I realized immediately that it gave me the ability to treat more proximal and more distal tibial fractures than the implant which I had been using. I scrubbed in with him on a couple of cases to learn the new techniques and I'm now happy with my own results."*

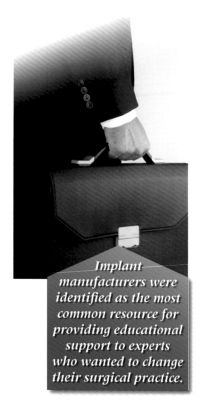

Implant manufacturers were identified as the most common resource for providing educational support to experts who wanted to change their surgical practice.

Two faculty members said that attending a trauma course had been their major learning resource in affecting a change in practice. Both surgeons referred to cadaveric dissections carried out on an educational course—one on a Master's course and one on a course on pelvis and acetabular surgery. Three surgeons felt that being a faculty member was their most important learning resource. As a faculty member, they were exposed to new ideas whilst attending a course and had the ability to discuss them with their peers and with the visiting experts. All three of the surgeons had identified faculty membership as being their most important learning resource in an earlier phase of the study.

Two surgeons said that their learning resources were journals, which they accessed online and one surgeon said that he had carried out his own clinical research. Two surgeons felt that they were able to affect the change by being self-taught and one surgeon admitted that he really was not able to identify what educational resources he had used to change his surgical technique.

As with all other groups who have been examined, clinical problems were the main reason for a change in surgical practice. Becoming aware of new technology was also critically important and many of the changes that were caused by clinical problems would not have occurred if new technology had not been available.

Surgeons who did make changes were heavily reliant on the educational support given to them by implant manufacturers in the form of technique guides, workshops, and visits from company representatives.

8.5   Summary

- Nearly every orthopedic surgeon changes an aspect of his practice every year.
- Two drivers exist for change at all stages in a surgeon's career—clinical problems and technological innovations.
- Numerous resources are used to help surgeons effect change but two—interpersonal interaction with colleagues and the use of manufacturers technique guides—are most commonly used.
- If change is driven by advances in technology then specific, non-CME accredited information provided by implant manufacturers is the preferred educational resource for surgeons at all stages in their careers.

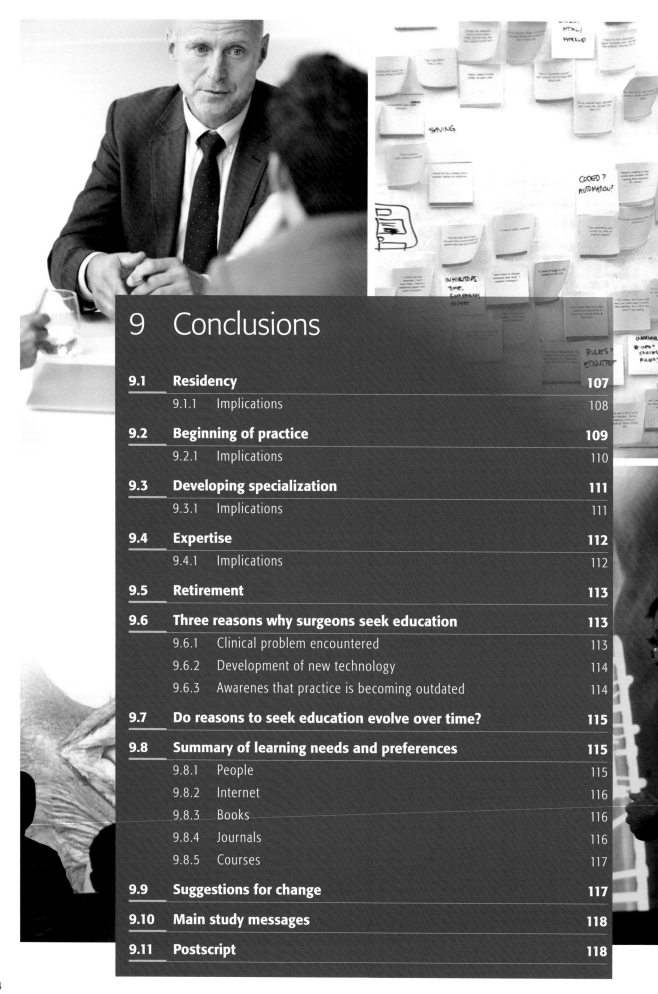

9 Conclusions

Chapter 9
Conclusions

The lifelong learning study used one-on-one discussion to gain insight into the evolution of surgeons' educational needs during the various stages of their careers. Over 65 hours of recorded interviews were collected and the 3500 questions asked to 147 surgeons informed this summary of responses. Numerous suggestions were made by the surgeons to improve educational offerings to better meet their needs.

With the introduction of new techniques and technologies the science of surgery is advancing every year. This inexorable march of progress means that surgeons need to continually evaluate their current practice and update it when needed. Patients, health care providers, and insurers expect that surgeons will educate themselves throughout their professional lives. Although experience is still a key factor associated with successful practice, patients now expect experience to be combined with the latest knowledge and skills. As a result lifelong learning is now part of surgical practice in most parts of the world and therefore educators need to serve all sections of the surgical community and not merely "surgeons-in-training" because the need to learn never stops throughout a surgical career.

Current medical education for surgeons seems not to have resulted in the changes that surgeons and their patients wish to see. [1–3] It is possible that part of this lack of success may be due to the failure of educators to understand how surgeons progress through their careers and how their learning needs and preferences change with time. Little is known about this subject [4–6] and this study attempts to explore these issues by listening to voices of surgeons.

The interpretation of any scientific study is problematic because all studies have their own limitations with regard to validity. In orthopedics and traumatology quantitative studies have problems with patient selection, outcome measures, and follow up. How many articles advocating a particular treatment have proved to be false as the accumulation of long-term data has shown original enthusiasm to be misplaced?

Qualitative studies like this one also have their own limitations. We cannot be sure that we asked the "right" questions to the "right" people. All the surgeons who were interviewed had some active connection with the sponsoring body. Moreover, they volunteered to give up some of their time to be interviewed. This group of surgeons therefore does not represent the "average" surgeon but a group of highly motivated health professionals who clearly had a pre-existing interest in education. Although surgeons were interviewed from all continents of the world, the largest country (Peoples Republic of China) was underrepresented due to communication and language issues.

That being said, the methodology used was reliable. Because the aim of the study was to explain a process and not to test or verify an existing theory, the use of the grounded theory approach of sociologists Glaser and Strauss (7) was fully justifiable.

Forty-seven surgeons were initially interviewed in both focus groups and individually before the main study instrument in accordance with grounded theory's iterative study design. Analysis of this preliminary data informed the design of the next cycle of data acquisition [8].

One hundred surgeons were interviewed in depth, half by telephone and half face-to-face. This number is larger than might be expected for such a study. A large number was chosen for two reasons. Firstly, there was substantial cultural background diversity and carrying out a smaller survey may have missed key cultural differences vital to the successful adaptation of educational programs to meet local needs.

The second reason for the size of the study relates to the interviewers them-selves. If a single or small group of highly trained individuals had carried out the interviews it might have been possible to have true cycles of simultaneous data collection and analysis leading to continual refining of the questions. This was not possible because surgeons and not educationalists carried out the interviews. It was felt that the advantage of surgeons talking to surgeons out-weighed the advantages of conducting a study on a smaller group of surgeons. Their stories were recorded, and individual reproduced in this monograph, to allow the variety of surgical experiences to be shared with the reader. No attempt was made to channel answers to reflect a particular viewpoint and the similarities and differences of the responses are the result of this process.

What is the best representation of learning over the span of a career?

The study reveals certain patterns of career development and the cultural differences that exist around the world. Understanding these stages and the changing educational requirements associated with each stage has implications for educators. As with all qualitative studies this chapter on conclusions will inevitably outline questions that were not answered and it is these questions that will set the agenda for subsequent studies.

Existing models of life and career pathways [9–14] suggest that distinct stages can be described within an individual's career.

Psychologist Daniel Levinson identified two types of stages—stable and transitional periods. Transitions occur as a man moved from one stable life stage to another. These transitions were frequently traumatic and if applied to medical careers would be expected to be times when a surgeon would need and seek additional educational support.

This study identified five distinct career or developmental stages that orthopedic surgeons pass through during their careers. Four of these five are directly relevant to educational organizations in terms of the education that they currently offer and will have to provide in the future. The study also identified transition points but these were very variable in their significance and were not usually associated with periods of intense stress. This finding does not, of course, invalidate Levinson's model because he was looking at the whole of a man's life rather than purely the stages in his career. Many surgeons experience transitions in their personal life, which may be both sudden and painful. These changes may interface with their careers and their ability to deliver top quality care but the interaction between personal and professional life was not examined in this study and may be an area for future research.

The five stages indentified in this study are outlined below.

9.1   Residency

Surgeons undergo a period of formal education, during which they practice under a degree of supervision. The period of formal training varies from 3 to 8 years in length. This stage is characterized by the presence of a formal curriculum and formal training pathways, although these are of varying significance in different parts of the world. Independent practice is usually not allowed and in most residency programs successful completion of a residency program involves passing a formal examination or set of formal examinations.

The variability in residency training is considerable around the world. Some residency programs are much shorter than others and when this occurs, surgeons who complete their residency training often undergo an additional period of supervised surgical practice within a teaching institution.

The degree of supervision also varies considerably in different parts of the world but there is an overall trend in the developed world towards greater supervision of a residents work particularly in the field of operative surgery. Although this increased degree of supervision may result in improved patient care, the amount of independent surgical experience is decreasing during residency making the transition from residency into independent practice potentially harder.

Although all the residency programs examined had formal curricula, nearly all the residents questioned said that their best learning experiences came from specific patients that they treated. Seeing a new patient, working that patient up, operating on them and following them up was by far the best way to learn—providing that their teaching institutions offered them adequate support and supervision throughout each part of the patient pathway. Elements of the traditional "apprenticeship" still survive and flourish today.

In the developed world and especially within the European Union [15] there is a move towards reducing the number of hours doctors work per week. This has resulted in a decrease in the exposure of trauma residents to certain types of patients, especially emergency cases. The combination of decreased working hours, decreasing numbers of patients treated, and increased supervision is resulting in the production of less experienced surgeons, although this may be at least partially offset by the increase in well organized teaching that is characteristic of many training schemes [16].

This stage in a surgeon's career corresponds in time to the entering adult world stage in Levinson's model [9]. It is indeed a time when the surgeon makes initial choices about his occupation.

Historically residency was designed to train "general orthopedic surgeons" who had sufficient training to allow them to safely practice orthopedics when entering independent practice. This cohort of surgeons entered independent practice as generalists and subsequently decided to specialize after a period of generalized practice. This study has shown that most current orthopedic trainees decide during residency which subspecialty they will enter and they begin their subspecialty training during residency, confirming the work of Ko et al. [17].

This finding differs from Nancy Bennett's model [11] of a surgeons career where the decision to subspecialize, or differentiate, is made following a period of independent practice where they are finding their feet and trying to conform. The time when surgeons decide to subspecialize also does not fit in well with Donald Supers [9–10] model of career development. Residency now appears to have elements from the first three stages of Super's model. It is certainly characterized by an individual's first introduction to work (Growth stage) but also has elements of the Exploration phase where individuals gather more specific information about themselves and the world of work and the establishment stage where individuals try to match their interests and capabilities to their occupation. Roger Rennekamp and Martha Nall's model [7–8] fits in best with this new pattern of residency. Their entry stage describes the reality of residency well but elements of the colleague stage are also now present in residency as the surgeon starts to build one area of expertise for which they are noted.

9.1.1   Implications

This study has shown that residency is changing to reflect the new realities of less time available for training, carried out with a greater degree of supervision. The implications for educational providers include the following:

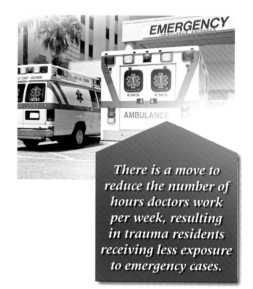

There is a move to reduce the number of hours doctors work per week, resulting in trauma residents receiving less exposure to emergency cases.

- Teaching organizations would appear to need to focus not only on providing information but also helping residents access relevant, valid, and significant information from the vast amount available online and from other channels.
- Teaching organizations need to consider adapting their current educational material to make it navigable and available online through small hand held devices.
- Faculty within teaching organizations may need faculty training programs to better prepare faculty to teach practical skills, provide consistent feedback on resident performance, and become effective mentors for their residents.
- Teaching organizations, hospitals, professional organizations, employers, and policy makers need to be aware that future young consultants will not have the same experience and skill mix of earlier times. These surgeons may require more support and their responsibilities may need to change to reflect their relative inexperience.

9.2 Beginning of practice

In this stage the surgeon moves from supervised practice to independent practice. Of all phases studied, this was the most variable in a surgeon's career. The length of time that the beginning of practice stage lasts varies between 1 and 5 years, depending on the degree of training and experience gained in residency.

Bennett's [14] model of a surgical career envisages a sudden change from supervised practice into independent practice. The stage is described as a desire by surgeons to learn how to carry out practice and find out what the norms of behavior are so that they can fit into their new work environment. When this occurs the transition from residency to independent practice is dramatic and very stressful to the surgeon. This pattern of career development is still seen in many countries, most notably in Great Britain and the United States of America but is becoming less common. This sudden transition stage correlates well with Levison's description of the age 30 transition and the beginning of practice stage fits in well with Super's establishment stage and Rennekamp and Nall's colleague stage.

A second career pathway is becoming more common. In this pathway the surgeon completes residency and then enters a period of supervised practice. This can take the form of a specialized fellowship where the fellow enjoys increasing independence over the period of the fellowship. Alternatively, surgeons may continue to work at their training institutes for many years with slowly decreasing levels of supervision.

There are significant cultural differences around the world. The English-speaking world traditionally had a sudden change from the end of residency to full independent practice. This is altering due to the reduced time for training in residency. More surgeons are taking fellowships or joining group practices where professional help is instantly available for clinical problems.

The German-speaking world maintains a strict hierarchical system with a single professor being responsible for his department in a hospital. This in turn means that most surgeons in Germany experience an extensive period of further training where their work is supervised after the completion of residency. Some surgeons never achieve full independent practice.

This study has shown the presence of two different transitions. Global teaching organizations need to understand the different career pathways and transitions to independent practice to more precisely target their educational offerings.

Although it would appear that the learning needs of these two career pathways should be radically different, the study has shown that both groups feel that interactivity with a senior surgeon is the most helpful educational resource available to them.

The study has shown that training in residency is changing due to decreased time available for training and increased supervision of a trainee's work. These factors are likely to increase in the future making a sudden transition into full independent practice harder and harder. One question for future study is how the start of independent practice can be modified to provide more support for surgeons. Although a mentoring system would appear to be a logical response, recent work has shown considerable hostility to a formal mentoring system, even though informal mentoring relationships are very helpful to surgeons at this stage of their careers [15].

9.2.1 Implications

The implications for educational providers include:
- Surgeons at this stage in their career value one-on-one discussion as their preferred method of learning and certain educational events, such as course and distance Internet-based learning, are often not best suited to this need.
- The commonest educational need expressed by this group of surgeons is the ability to talk with seniors about their clinical problems. Interactivity and discussion is most valued by this group. Facilitation of such interactions would appear to be a logical educational strategy.
- The vast majority of these interactions occur within the institution in which surgeons are working. Teaching surgeons in independent practice how to act as effective coaches to their younger colleagues may well make such interactions more successful.
- Senior or peer advice may not always be available within a single institution. To bypass this, educational organizations could facilitate the creation of Internet-based communities of practice, which allow interaction between surgeons from different hospitals.

9.3 Developing specialization

This stage in a surgeon's career is the time when the surgeon starts to specialize. This study has shown that two career pathways exist with regard to developing a specialist interest. The commonest pathway in the developed world is for the surgeon to begin developing a specialist interest while in residency [16]. Most residency programs rotate their trainees through the various subspecialties of orthopedics and trauma. Residents usually decide on their specialty interests during these rotations and often arrange their rotations to maximize their exposure to training. These surgeons then frequently arrange to take a fellowship in their chosen subspecialty. The decision to specialize is taken much earlier than used to be the case and the transition to specialty training is, therefore, much more gradual and controlled than in the past. The decision to specialize in a particular field is influenced by many factors but the presence of a role model or mentor seems very important to many surgeons [18].

In the developing world the decision to subspecialize is often taken much later in a surgeon's career, usually at a time when the surgeon is in independent practice. This pattern of career development closely follows Bennett's (14) description of stage two of her career model, where instead of surgeons trying to find out what the norms of behavior are and trying to fit in, they start to try to differentiate their practice from their colleagues.

The educational needs of these two groups are different. Those surgeons who decide to specialize early have their initial training within an established teaching institute. Educational resources are available and training programs exist. For those who start later no such programs exist and the surgeon must be more active in searching out suitable educational resources.

Although the learning needs of the two groups are different, both groups report that their best learning experiences were those which involved interaction with seniors or peers. This preference is identical to that shown by surgeons who are just starting their surgical practice.

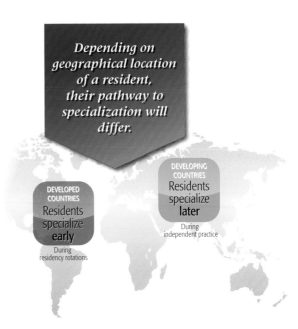

9.3.1 Implications

The implications for a teaching organization include:

- Events targeted to surgeons who wish to develop a specialist interest will need to take into account that two disparate groups of surgeons will be interested in attending. Junior surgeons will have back-up within their teaching institute and may well have a mentor/advisor to help them after the event. More senior surgeons, especially those working in a community hospital, will have none of these additional resources available to them.
- Following an educational event or program, senior surgeons may well need to carry out the procedures described on their own. This is unlikely to occur with the more junior group. The seniors may require post-event support, perhaps in the form of instant access to teaching material used, at their time of need.

- Most surgeons value interactivity with peers or seniors as their best learning experience. Teaching organizations can facilitate this in a variety of ways, such as communities of practice. Those organizations who run educational events should be aware that faculty membership is felt to be the best learning experience enjoyed by surgeons largely because of this interactivity.

9.4   Expertise

This stage of a surgeon's career occurs when the surgeon becomes the acknowledged expert in his or her field of expertise. He or she frequently provides a secondary or even tertiary referral service. Within the medical community in which the surgeon operates, he or she is regarded as the acknowledged expert. The surgeon is frequently involved in teaching both formally and informally.

The study has shown that nearly every senior surgeon who was interviewed had expertise in a given subspecialty. Although these surgeons functioned as experts many of them did not recognize that they were the local experts. Many felt that they would always continue to learn and improve and that there was never an end point to their practice. Although these surgeons appear to fit in with Super's [6] maintenance stage of a career, they differ significantly from that model in as much as they seem to be continually exploring new avenues and continuing to develop their own clinical skills. This difference could at least be partially explained by the fact that Super concentrated on the corporate world and not the world of the professional.

Regardless of specialty, or country of practice, most experts commented that they still prefer to acquire knowledge and skills by interacting with their peers. Opportunities to do so are limited for experts, especially those working in smaller hospitals where true peers do not exist. Their typical form of learning is learning by experience, but they much prefer to discuss cases on a one–to-one basis.

Nearly all the experts who were also faculty members on educational courses rated their faculty membership as being their best learning experience. Faculty members value the incentive to get up-to-date when asked to prepare presentations and relish interactivity with their peers that occurs during an educational event. When faculty training occurs this too is rated very highly by experts as a learning experience. Some surgeons who are not faculty members obtain their peer interaction by attending national or international conferences.

9.4.1   Implications
Implications for a teaching organization include:
- Because surgeons report that they never stop learning it would appear that education appears to be vital for all surgeons even those considered to be experts or key opinion leaders.

- Faculty membership is the most valued educational resource for expert surgeons. Medical educators could consider enhancing the learning experiences of their faculty by ensuring that more opportunities for interaction are given to faculty, possibly in the form of case-based interactive discussions for faculty only
- Faculty development programs are also potent potential vehicles for facilitating learning in this expert group. Faculty development appears not only to produce better teachers for the benefit of the whole medical community, but also facilitates learning by experts because of a greater understanding of what makes effective and ineffective learning.

9.5   Retirement

The beginning of this stage may occur when the surgeon first starts to think about retirement. This may occur at a comparatively young age. The stage is characterized by Bennett [14] as a stage when there is a relative freeze in professional development. Learning may still occur as a result of clinical need. This stage of a surgeons career was not formally examined in this study, although some surgeons who were interviewed fell into this career stage. No valid conclusions can therefore be drawn and a formal examination of the learning needs of this group may form part of a further study.

9.6   Three reasons why surgeons seek education

The study identified three main reasons why surgeons look for education. These educational drivers are identical to those described by Robert Fox et al in their book, *Changing and Learning in the lives of Physicians [20].*

Although these three drivers can be identified and defined, a surgeon's decision to seek educational help often involves more than one factor. Surgeons may continue to practice in one way for many years even though they know that the clinical results are not as good as they or their patients would wish. New technology is then developed and the surgeon becomes aware of its presence and its potential. Because a solution to his patient's problems may now be available, the surgeon reassesses his results and what previously was acceptable now becomes a clinical issue that needs to be addressed.

9.6.1   Clinical problem encountered
This is by far the commonest reason for surgeons to look for educational support. This driver occurs at all stages of a surgical career.

There are two common ways in which clinical problems cause a surgeon to look for educational help. The first occurs when a surgeon comes across an unusual case for the first time and does not know exactly how to best handle the situation. The second occurs when a surgeon treats a patient in a standard way and then encounters an unforeseen complication.

The characteristics of this type of need are that it is unpredictable, ie, the surgeon cannot know when an individual case or complication will occur. Therefore, a vital characteristic of the education required is that it must be available instantly or within a very short period of time to give surgeons help when they and their patients need it.

Modalities suitable to fill these needs include Internet access to relevant information but most surgeons prefer the opportunity to discuss the case with a peer or expert. Teaching organizations would appear to have opportunities to facilitate both forms of learning by addressing the issues of getting the surgeon to the relevant information needed and facilitating interaction, either by creating communities of practice or by improving coaching and feedback skills through faculty development programs.

9.6.2   Development of new technology

This is the second commonest reason why surgeons seek educational support. This driver occurs at all stages of a surgical career. Trauma surgery is characterized by the rapid evolution of new surgical implants and techniques. When surgeons become aware of these advances they frequently wish to access education to allow them to use the new implants. Such education needs are not as urgent as those that arise from clinical issues and needs are often dominated by the acquisition of new mechanical skills rather than new judgment pathways.

Educational organizations can facilitate learning new techniques and technology in a variety of ways. The key messages given by the surgeons who took part in this study is that they need to acquire technical skills when introduction of new technology is the educational driver. They do not seem to feel that a fully evidence-based, balanced teaching program is required to achieve this. What they want is education more focused on acquiring the relevant skills. Implant manufacturers provide such programs and these non-CME programs seem valued by surgeons even though they are often product and not evidence-based.

9.6.3   Awarenes that practice is becoming outdated

If a surgeon becomes aware that his or her practice is getting out-of-date this need for education characteristically occurs during the latter stages of a surgeon's career. Surgeons may become aware that younger surgeons have been appointed and have brought with them new techniques. Alternatively, surgeons may start to notice that their patients are not doing as well as others. This could perhaps be reflected in an increased inpatient stay for standard procedures. This educational need creeps up on a surgeon over a period of time. Surgeons are usually unaware of any potential issues of suboptimal performance until a clinical issue occurs.

The development of revalidation as a concept may bring these issues to the surface at a much earlier stage than currently occurs in most medical communities. The learning need is more complex than with the other two drivers since deficits usually exist not only in terms of knowledge and judgment but also in skills.

9.7 Do reasons to seek education evolve over time?

The study has given contradictory answers to the question of whether surgeons change the reasons why they look for education depending on their career level. Clinical problems and new technology are reasons why surgeons look for education at all career stages but other less important reasons are more specific to certain career stages.

In residency, passing examinations is a major educational driver and this occurs in no other stage of a surgeon's career. Similarly, preparation to give a presentation at a hospital meeting is very important in residency and only occurs rarely outside this stage. However, preparation for other presentations occurs at all career stages and more senior surgeons often require access to educational support to help them prepare for teaching assignments.

9.8 Summary of learning needs and preferences

9.8.1 People

Motivation to look for education may be fairly uniform among surgeons at all stages of their careers but the study clearly shows that surgeons differ markedly in their choice of preferred educational channels depending on their career stage.

Interaction with people is critically important for all surgeons. Residents value these interactions most of which occur with their attendings/consultants. Surgeons at the start of their careers are the group who report being most dependent on help and advice from colleagues. Many surgeons describe close, mentoring type relationships with a single named surgeon which were very helpful to them. Curiously, none of these relationships was a result of a formal mentoring process. This finding supports the meta-analysis carried out by doctor Dario Sambunjak [21] who reported that formal mentorship was found to be surprisingly uncommon even though mentorship was identified as an important influence on personal development and career guidance.

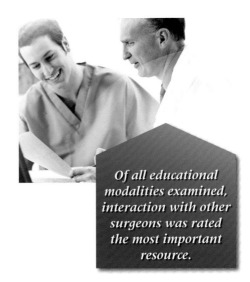

Of all educational modalities examined, interaction with other surgeons was rated the most important resource.

As the surgeon progresses, interactions with people seem to become more difficult to achieve. But when senior surgeons are able to interact with their peers, for example when they are acting as faculty on an educational congress or course, they rate these interactions as being their most effective educational resource. These findings would suggest that educational providers could focus on the facilitation of collegial interaction for surgeons, an idea, which is supported by the work of health policy researcher Anna Gagliardi et al. [22].

9.8.2   Internet

Use of the Internet is very popular at all stages of a surgeon's career but residents are the group who are most likely to request more and/or different Internet-based services.

Existing Internet resources are criticized by all for several reasons. There is, if anything, too much information available online. Existing search engines are not specific enough to meet the clinical needs of the surgeons who use them. They do not differentiate between valid and invalid information nor can they rate the importance or otherwise of a given piece of information. These findings exactly match those of Bennett et al. [23].

Residents are used to access information via apps on their mobile devices. They request the same service from educational providers. They would like clinically relevant information to be available whenever and wherever they need it. Such an informational package should also include appropriate navigation to allow the surgeon rapid access to the information needed to help a patient.

Residents also request that existing educational events have post-event material available online to act as reminders.

ELearning does not feature significantly in the learning portfolio of any of the groups studied but some residents comment on the lack of available material. This finding differs from that of Assistant Professor and Associate Director of Continuing Medical Education, University of Alabama School of Medicine Dr Linda Casebeer [24], who found over 100,000 US physicians had taken part in Internet-based CME activities. This could reflect a lack of suitable material in the field of orthopedics and trauma or could reflect an unwillingness of this group of surgeons to use such resources. This study cannot answer this question and this may be a subject for further research.

> *Courses in orthopedic trauma are most valued by residents and surgeons in the very early stages of their careers; senior surgeons find existing courses do not meet their needs.*

9.8.3   Books

Books are mainly used by residents. They buy books early in their careers and tend to buy a small number of "classical" texts. Initially they read these books on a chapter-by-chapter basis but very quickly they start to use small sections of books that relate to the clinical issues that they face. The pattern of use is identical for print and electronic versions of a book.

As surgeons become more senior and more specialized, their use of books declines markedly. Specialized textbooks are criticized as being rapidly out of date. Expert surgeons rarely use books preferring instead to access information from journal articles via the Internet.

9.8.4   Journals

Journal articles are used as educational resources by surgeons at all levels of seniority. The pattern of use has changed with the passage of time. Journals used to be bought and read cover to cover. Today the need and demand for journal articles is as great if not greater than ever, but the need to access and read the whole journal is much less than it was. Journal articles are read by accessing them through the Internet using a search engine. This clearly has implications for producers of journals.

9.8.5   Courses

Existing educational courses in the field of orthopedic trauma seem to be valued mainly by residents and surgeons at a very early stage of their careers. More senior surgeons feel that existing formal courses do not meet their educational needs, which are largely focused on the clinical problems they see. Those surgeons who are currently at the expert stage in their careers grew up with courses as part of their educational portfolio. Many expert surgeons feel that new courses could be designed for them. They reject existing course formats but wish to create new ones.

9.9   Suggestions for change

Most surgeons value their current and past educational resources however, many feel that there are gaps in currently available educational resources. Their suggestions for change include:

- Intelligent search engines which take surgeons to relevant selected information targeted to their needs.
- Navigated educational resources available on mobile devices that take the surgeon rapidly to solutions for the clinical problem faced.
- Online resources for residents focused on their need to pass examinations.
- Navigable Internet access to all course material used at educational courses after the event.
- Development of short educational events targeted to specific clinical problems for surgeons in practice. Such events would clearly require a rigorous needs assessment. Participants would be peers, the faculty would be experts, and the format would be largely interactive.
- Creation of short-term fellowships for surgeons in practice focused on a single pathology/treatment strategy. Fellowships have been shown to be highly effective as an educational event [25].
- Development of forums where peers could exchange information and experiences. This could be achieved either by enhancing face-to-face contact at existing educational events or congresses by the creation of online communities of practice.

9.10   Main study messages

The lifelong learning study involved 147 surgeons answering over 3500 questions. Over 65 hours of interviews were recorded. A large number of themes were explored. It is clearly impossible to condense all this data into key conclusions without the danger of omission, but the following five points seem, in the minds of the authors, to be the main messages of the study.

- Surgeons progress through definable stages in their careers. The nature of these stages, and the transitions that accompany them, change with time. Marked cultural differences exist.
- Although two reasons for accessing educational help—clinical problems and new technology—occur at all career stages, the preferred method of accessing educational help changes with the stage of a surgeon's career.
- The advent of the Internet has completely changed the way in which all surgeons access information, but there remains huge problems in ensuring that surgeons can access the information they actually need rapidly through the Internet. Existing search engines do not seem fit for this purpose.
- New technologies have changed the way in which surgeons learn but talking cases over with peers or seniors is still the best learning experience for most surgeons.
- Faculty membership is a powerful learning experience for many surgeons. Faculty development can further enhance the learning experience inherent in being a teacher.

9.11   Postscript

The authors hope that this monograph may stimulate educators and surgeons alike to try new ways of educating surgeons to reflect their career stage and that this in turn may result in improved patient care.

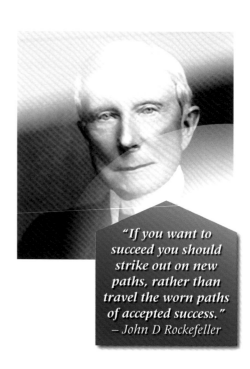

"If you want to succeed you should strike out on new paths, rather than travel the worn paths of accepted success."
– John D Rockefeller

Bibliography

1. **Institute of Medicine** (2000) "To Err Is Human: Building a Safer Health System". *The National Academies Press.*

2. **Charatan F** (2000) "Clinton acts to reduce medical mistakes". *BMJ Publishing Group.* doi:10.1136/bmj.320.7235.597.

3. **Weingart SN, Wilson RM, Gibberd RW, et al** (March 2000) "Epidemiology of medical error". *BMJ;* 320 (7237):774–777.

4. **Teunissen PW, Doman T (**2008) Lifelong learning at work: *BMJ;* 336:667

5. **Dale V, Pierce S E, Stephen A** (2009) May Surgeons views about—and participation in—lifelong learning. Summary Report, January 2009. www.live.ac.uk/documents/VetCPD_

6. **Shaughnessy AF, Slawson DC** (1999) Are we providing doctors with the training and tools for lifelong learning. *BMJ;* 319:1280

7. **Glaser B, Strauss A** (1967) The discovery of grounded theory: strategies for qualitative research Chicago: Aldine

8. **Kennedy T, Lingard L** (2006) Making sense of grounded theory Med Educ; 40:101–108

9. **Levinson DJ** (1978) Seasons of a man's life. New York: Ballantaine Books.

10. **Rennekamp RA, Nall M** (1994) Growing through the stages: A new look at professional growth *Journal of Extension;* Vol 32 (1).

11. **Rennekamp RA, Nall M** Professional growth; a guide for professional development. Lexington: University of Kentucky Cooperative Extension Service.

12. **Super DE** (1957) The psychology of careers. New York: Harper and Row.

13. **Super DE**, Self concepts in vocational development in DE Super (ed), Career development: Self concept theory New York ; College Entrance Examination Board.

14. **Bennett NL** (1990) Theories of Adult Development for Continuing Education. *J Cont Educ Health Prof;* 10(2): 167–175.

15. European working time directive http://www.direct.gov.uk/en/Employment/Employees/WorkingHoursAndTimeOff/DG_10029426

16. http://www.mee.nhs.uk/our_work/work_priorities/review_of_ewtd__impact_on_tra.aspx

17. **Ko CY, Whang EE, Karamanoukian R, et al** (1998) What is the best method of surgical training? A report of America's leading senior surgeons. *Arch. Surg;* 133 (8):900–905.

18. **McKinstry B, Macnicol M, Elliot K, et al** (2005) The transition from learner to provider/teacher: The learning needs of new orthopaedic consultants. *BMC Med Educ;* 5:17.

19. **McCord JH, McDonald R, Sippel RS, et al** (2009) Surgical career choices: The vital impact of mentoring. *J Surg Res Jul;* 155(1):136–141.

20. **Fox RD, Mazmanian PE, Purnam RW** (1989) Changing and learning in the lives of Physicians. New York: Praeger.

21. **Sambunjak D, Straus SE** (2006) Marusic Mentoring in academic medicine: a systematic review. *JAMA;* 296(9):1103–1115.

22. **Gagliardi AR, Wright FC, Anderson MA, et al** (2007) The role of collegial interaction in continuing professional development. *J Contin Educ Health Prof;* 27(4):214–219.

23. **Bennett NL, Casebeer LL, Zheng S, et al** (2006) Information–seeking behaivours and reflective practice. *J Contin Educ Health Prof;* 26 (2):120–127.

24. **Casebeer L, Engler S, Bennett N, et al** (2008) A controlled trial of the effectiveness of Internet continuing medical education. *BMC Med;* 6:37.

25. **Lown BA, Newman LR, Hatem CJ** (2009) The personal and professional impact of a fellowship in medical education. *Acad Med;* 84(8):1089–1097

26. **Fox RD, Bennett NL** (1998) Learning and change: implications for continuing medical education. *BMJ;* 316(7129):466–468. Review

The authors

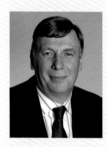

Piet de Boer

Piet de Boer was educated at Downing College Cambridge and St Thomas' Hospital London. In 1985 he became a consultant Orthopedic Surgeon in York, UK. He was the first director of education for the AO Foundation in Davos Switzerland. Author of four successful books in the fields of orthopedics and medical education he currently runs his own education company.

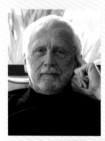

Robert D Fox

Robert D Fox has authored or coauthored four books including the study *Changing and Learning in the Lives of Physicians, The Physician as Learner, The Continuing Professional Development of Physicians: Integrating Theory and Practice* with D Davis and B Barnes, and the book length report of the IOM, *Redesigning Continuing Education in the Health Professions* (coauthored with a panel of experts). He has authored or coauthored more than 100 articles, book chapters, papers, and invited presentations or addresses to national and international organizations. He served as editor of the Journal of Continuing Education in the Health Professions. In a University of Wisconsin study of most important books and journals in CME, his first three books were ranked 1 through 3 by a forty- member panel of his peers. Currently he is professor emeritus of Educational Leadership and Policy Studies at the University of Oklahoma and is senior consultant to Professional Development Associates in Florida.

Copyright © 2012
by AO Foundation
Stettbachstrasse 6
8600 Dübendorf
Switzerland

Appendix I

Interview template for main study

Question 1A
How would you describe the current stage in your career?

Question 1B
Do you recognize there have been different stages in your career? If so, how would you describe them?

Question 2
Can you remember particular methods of learning that were characteristic of Stage 1—Residency?

- What role did peers play?

- What role did literature play (eg, books, journals)?

- What role did formal educational events such as AO courses play in your education?

- What role did Internet resources play? What resources have you used (eg, AO/Google/PubMed)?

- What role did hospital meetings, such as morbidity and mortality, play?

- When looking back, which method of learning was most important during residency?

Question 3
Can you remember particular methods of learning that were characteristic of Stage 2—Beginning practice?

- What role did peers play?

- What role did literature play (eg, books, journals)?

- What role did formal educational programs play (AO and other courses)?

- What role did Internet resources play? What resources have you used (eg, AO/Google/PubMed)?

- What role did hospital meetings, such as morbidity and mortality, play?

- When looking back, which method of learning was most important at the beginning of independent practice?

Question 4
Can you remember particular methods of learning that were characteristic of Stage 3—Increasing specialization?

Did trauma become your major interest? Yes/No
If yes—how did you learn about trauma? If not, how did you learn about your chosen specialty?

- What role did peers play?

- What role did formal educational programs play (AO and other courses)?

- How important was faculty experience in- and outside of the AO Foundation?

- What role did literature play (eg, books, journals)?

- What role did Internet resources play? What resources have you used (eg, AO/Google/PubMed)?

- What role did hospital meetings, such as morbidity and mortality, play?

- Thinking back, which method of learning was most important during Stage 3, when you began increasing your specialization?

Question 5
Over time, has trauma become more important, less important, or maintained the same importance in your practice?

How do you keep up-to-date with trauma management?

- What role did/do formal educational programs play (AO and other courses)?

- How important was/is faculty experience in- and outside of the AO Foundation?

- What role did/does literature play (eg, books, journals)?

- What role did/do Internet resources play? What resources have you used (eg, AO/Google/PubMed)?

- What role did/do hospital meetings, such as morbidity and mortality, play?

- Which method of learning is currently most important for you?

Question 6
In the last year, have you made any changes to the way you practice trauma surgery?

What did you change and why?

In what way(s) did learning play a role in changing your practice? What learning resources did you use?

Did AOTrauma play a role in changing your practice and if so, how?

Are you an AO Alumni or AOTrauma faculty?
If so, what is your role and why did you join?

If the AO could do one thing to improve the care you give to patients what would that be?